Love Your Age

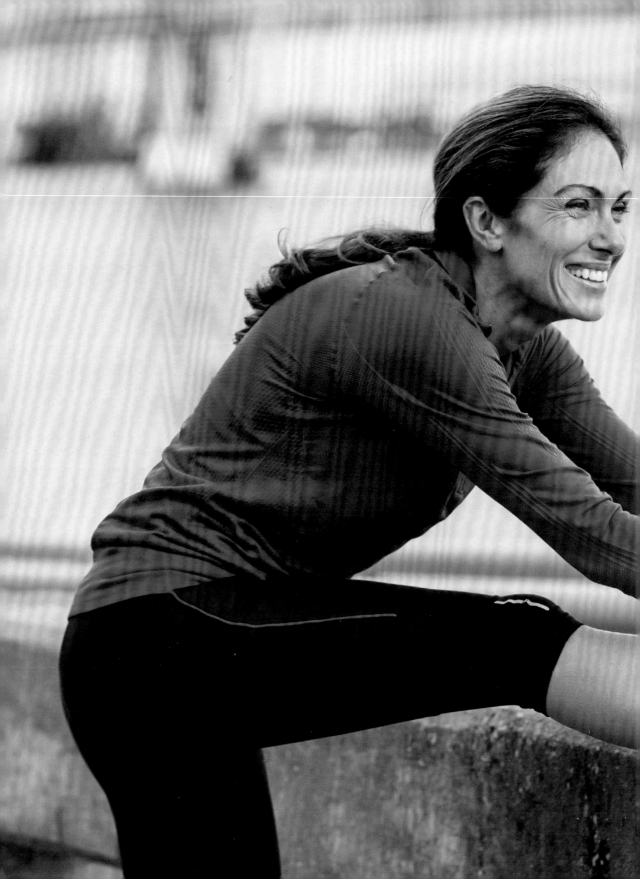

Love
Your Age

THE SMALL-STEP
SOLUTION TO A
better, longer,
happier life

BARBARA HANNAH GRUFFERMAN

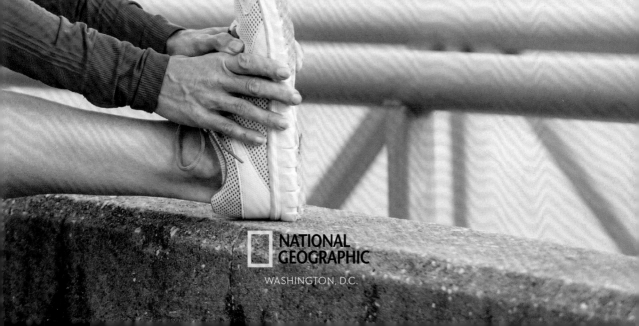

NATIONAL
GEOGRAPHIC

WASHINGTON, D.C.

Since 1888, the National Geographic Society has funded more than 12,000 research, exploration, and preservation projects around the world. National Geographic Partners distributes a portion of the funds it receives from your purchase to National Geographic Society to support programs including the conservation of animals and their habitats.

National Geographic Partners
1145 17th Street NW
Washington, DC 20036-4688 USA

Become a member of National Geographic and activate your benefits today at natgeo.com/jointoday.

For information about special discounts for bulk purchases, please contact National Geographic Books Special Sales: specialsales@natgeo.com

For rights or permissions inquiries, please contact National Geographic Books Subsidiary Rights: bookrights@natgeo.com

ISBN: 978-1-4262-1832-3

Printed in China

17/RRDS/1

To Sarah and Elizabeth, my daughters.
To all women, everywhere.

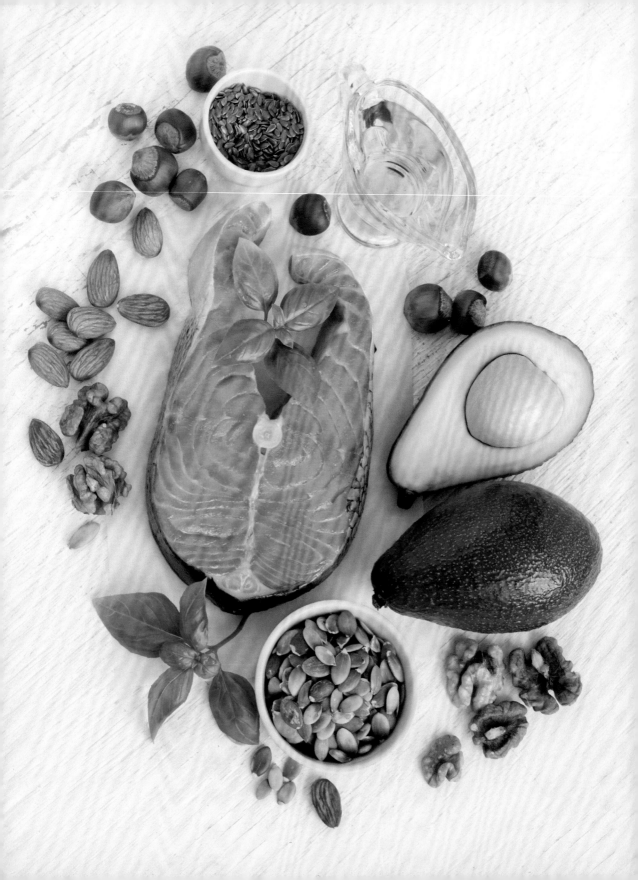

CONTENTS

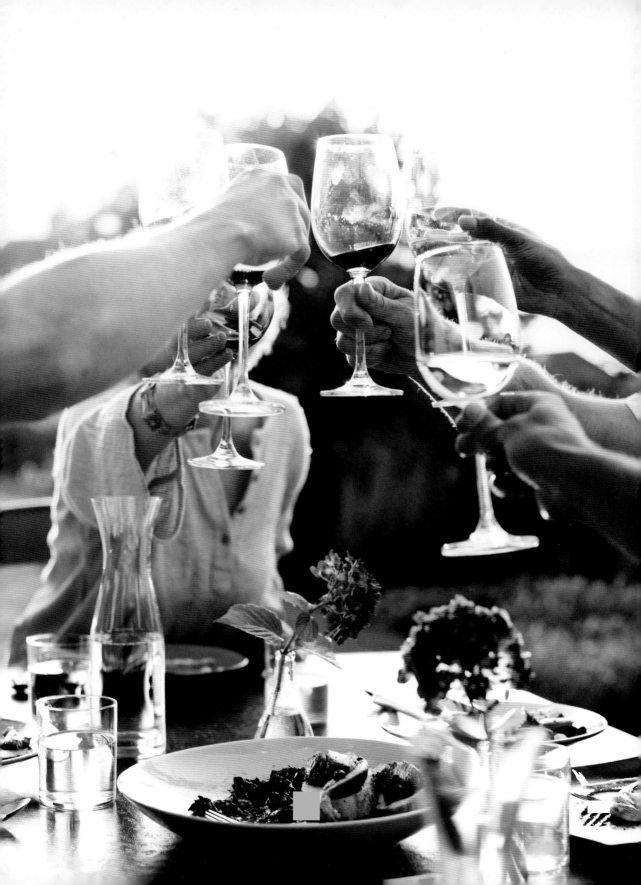

How One Small Step Sparked a Whole New Life

Several years ago, I stood on First Avenue with my two daughters and my husband, a few friends and neighbors, and lots of strangers. It was a glorious fall day, and we were watching packs of runners go by, caught up in the excitement of the New York City Marathon.

But despite the beauty of the day, all I could think about was how far I felt from the determined athletes passing just a few feet away. Unlike them, I was at one of the lowest points of my life. Facing 50 and not exactly loving this new age, I was feeling sluggish, slow, low-energy, and anything but strong and ambitious. I didn't like how my clothes fit or how my hair and skin looked. Having just packed on a few new menopausal pounds didn't help, but neither did the fact that I wasn't doing anything about it.

Stuck in my personal pity party, I watched the runners—especially those over 40—with amazement. I was filled with wonder about how anyone could run 26.2 miles. I couldn't even imagine walking that far ... or wanting to. Running represented only dreaded memories of Field Day in elementary school. It was like those runners and I were entirely different species.

Lost in my negativity, I was surprised when my younger daughter suddenly blurted, "One day I want to hold up a sign that says 'Go, Mom, Go!!'" Everyone stared at her. Then, as if on cue, they all turned and stared at me. My older daughter looked doubtful. My husband looked amused. I probably looked trapped. Feeling simultaneously horrified (really, what *was* she thinking?) and weirdly excited, I paused and said, "I don't know how, and I don't know when. But I will run this race. I promise."

On that day, which was immediately scorched into my memory bank of pivotal events, I vowed to make some changes—one small step at a time.

Still skeptical about running but inspired by my daughter's outburst, I looked for a program that didn't seem too intimidating for an out-of-shape woman in her late

40s. After spending a bit of time on the Internet, I discovered running expert Jeff Galloway's Run Walk Run program, which (as you might have guessed) alternates running and walking throughout the course of a workout.

"Okay," I thought. "I think I can manage that."

To ease into it, I started by simply taking walks every day, slowly making them both longer and faster. After a few weeks, I added some jogging. Not much at first—but eventually I worked up to a fifty-fifty split between running and walking.

My routine was simple but steadfast: On Mondays, Wednesdays, and Fridays, after I got the family out the door and before I started my workday, I'd don my running clothes, tie up my sneakers, pop in some earbuds, head to Central Park, and run (well, run/walk/run). My routine varied only to the extent that I sometimes spent a little more time running than walking—or vice versa, depending on my mood, the temperature, and which Tom Petty song was playing.

I couldn't have imagined it at the time, but choosing to adopt that one simple habit of running three times a week—rain or shine, all year long—became the foundation of a whole new life. I think the key was that once I decided to do it, I didn't look back. Running became nonnegotiable, and I realized that nothing else was so important that it couldn't be accomplished after my run or on my days off. And then something magical happened: My one new habit led to others.

• I ATE BETTER. Once I started getting regular physical exercise, I was inspired to fuel my body with better food, resulting in more energy, lost pounds, and improved over-all health. I reconsidered every meal and slowly gravitated away from takeout and packaged foods and toward home-cooked veggies, legumes, and healthy proteins. Since I was paying more attention to how my body felt, I noticed that big portions, fried foods, and sweets didn't sit very well. So I cut back on them and got into the habit of eating smaller meals throughout the day, which lessened food cravings and kept my blood sugar levels stable.

• I SLEPT MORE. Because I was more active during the day, I was more tired at night. This simple shift caused me to go to sleep earlier, and to sleep better and longer, which, in turn, helped me feel more alert, upbeat, and energetic than I'd been in years.

• I GOT STRONGER. I became interested in strengthening my body so I could be a more powerful runner, and created a daily habit of doing push-ups, planks, and squats. My muscle tone firmed up and my entire body looked and felt younger.

HOW ONE SMALL STEP SPARKED A WHOLE NEW LIFE

• I STOOD TALLER. Feeling stronger inside and out resulted in a dramatic increase in my self-esteem. I became more aware of my posture and body language. Both reflected a woman who was much more comfortable in her own skin (and clothes).

As each small step built on the last, I realized that my former grumpy, frumpy, lumpy state of being wasn't the inevitable result of getting older. It was the inevitable result of continuing to make the same unhealthy choices I'd been making for years.

Choices like putting everyone else first so that I felt perpetually stressed, rushed, and overwhelmed. And these feelings led me to other choices, like driving instead of walking (I'm in a hurry!), bingeing on Netflix instead of turning in early (I just need to decompress!), grabbing fast food instead of cooking (told you, I'm in a hurry!) … and on and on. All these little seemingly insignificant choices had turned into habits that had commandeered my life—and, worse, that were aging me prematurely.

But once my running habit snowballed into a better diet, sleep, and attitude, it was as if the clock started turning backward. I lost weight, found my waistline again, had more enthusiasm and better skin—and I smiled much, much more. I made a lot of new friends along the way, helping me to create a community of like-minded people. Thanks to my daughter's crazy idea, I'd finally gotten inspired to swap my "get old fast" mode for new "live better longer" habits—and they were working!

I know I'm not alone in having built up bad habits over the years. We all have them, and some might have even worked for us in the past. But the truth is that many of us are doing things every single day that are undermining the very things we want out of our lives: to feel healthy, happy, and productive for as long as possible.

Why do we do this? Usually because we don't recognize the problem, are afraid to change, or don't know how to make choices that are a better match for us now.

I'm living proof that the little steps we take every day don't stand alone: They all combine to determine how good we'll feel today, tomorrow, and in five years. In other words, we need to invest in ourselves *now* to have the life we want *later.* While it's never too early—or too late!—to let healthy habits into your life, you have to choose them over and over again every single day. That's how the small steps add up.

And building these habits doesn't need to be a huge ordeal! You don't need a live-in chef to eat more fruits and vegetables or a personal trainer to exercise more, or a professional stylist to overhaul your wardrobe. What you do need is information and inspiration (and maybe just a little nagging)—which is why I wrote this book.

But the most important tool for taking better care of yourself is in your own hands.

Human nature dictates that we are more secure in our comfort zones. But there's a huge difference between "secure" and "stuck." So if you're stuck in a place that just doesn't feel right anymore, you get to choose every day whether to perpetuate the same habits that are keeping you glued there—or take the steps to set yourself free.

Here's the best news: Even if you've been doing everything wrong (doubtful), most of our patterns are easy to fix. Every single step you take will make a difference in **how much you enjoy your life, how much you embrace who you are now, and how much you love your age.** The more steps you take, the bigger the difference.

For myself, after I took that first small step toward taking better care of myself, my life changed forever. I was physically, emotionally, and spiritually recharged.

But one of the most important results was that I fulfilled the promise I made to my daughter. After a few years of building my health, strength, and stamina, I felt ready to do the very thing I never thought I could: run all 26.2 miles of the New York City Marathon ... and enjoy every step of the way.

I never felt more proud or powerful than I did that day. Until I did it again a few years later ... And then again a few years after that.

Who knows? Maybe running marathons has gotten to be a habit ...

Don't Just Read This Book: Use It!

This book is all about the small choices we make—how they affect us and how we can change the results by changing our choices. Some of the suggestions will make you feel more confident. Some will make you stronger. Many will add joy to your days (and spark to your nights!). A few might even save your life. **All will no doubt help you feel good about your age, whatever it is.** You probably know some of this information already, but a little reminder never hurts. You can choose to keep what works for you, and skip the rest. The suggestions that help you the most will be the ones you adopt as a new routine—hopefully for a lifetime. But just the act of controlling your habits will get you back to being who you are truly meant to be: a woman who has every reason to **love yourself, love your life, and love your age.**

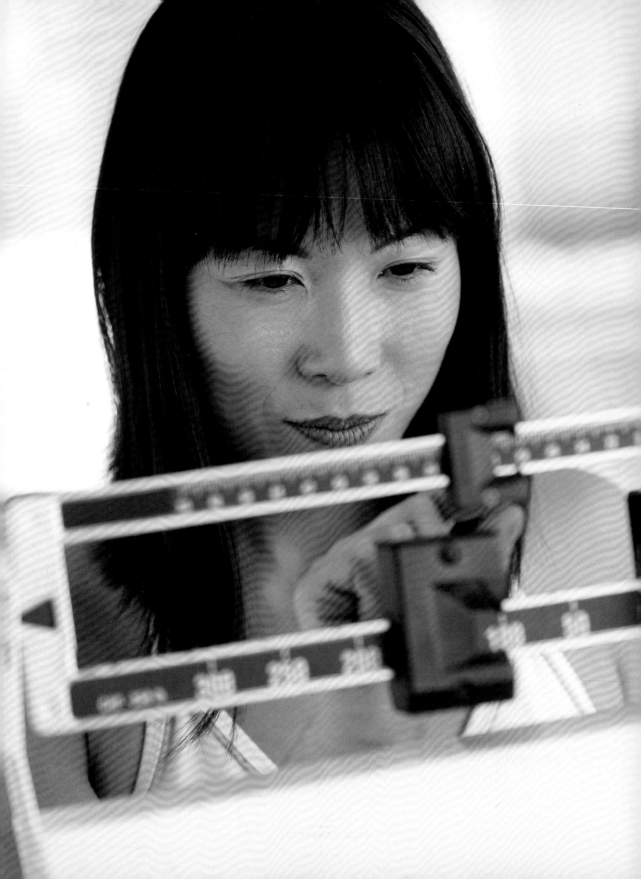

CHAPTER 1

Health Check-In

"The doctor of the future will give no medicine but will interest his or her patients in the care of the human frame, proper diet, and in the cause and prevention of disease."

—THOMAS EDISON

I've got a little mantra for you. Ready? Repeat after me:

"We can't control getting older, but we *can* control how we do it."

What does that mean? Well, after writing about positive aging for more than a decade, it's become clear to me that the path to a good, long life is pretty straightforward. What's more, like most paths, it's made up of a series of small steps. There is no fountain of youth, but you can help yourself feel great for longer, look great for longer, and probably even live longer if you:

- Put your well-being first.
- Maintain a healthy weight.
- Move your body.
- Make sleep a priority.
- Choose foods that nourish your body.
- Sustain a strong social network.
- Get regular health checks.
- Stay current with vaccines.
- Don't smoke.
- No, seriously—don't smoke.

Do you see the common denominator here? All of these are in your control. All of them.

Want to enjoy life at any age? Make health your #1 priority.

It's as simple as that.

It's hard—maybe even impossible—to have a vital life if you ignore your health. How you define "a vital life" is totally up to you. But whatever you love to do— whether it's teaching, fishing, painting, running a business, or running marathons—the first step to making your life better, richer, and very possibly longer is to focus on your health. And here's the bottom-line secret to healthy aging: Instead of hoping you can fix problems *after* they appear, focus on preventing them *before* they do.

Goal: Don't Go Before Your Time

Healthy aging isn't about avoiding death. (*News flash:* That's not an option.) It's about keeping our quality of life as high as possible for as long as possible and avoiding premature decline and death from preventable diseases.

Longevity experts call this approach "lengthening your health span," and generally have identified three hallmarks of successful aging:

❶ **Avoid succumbing to disease and disability.**
❷ **Sustain a high level of cognitive and physical functioning.**
❸ **Stay engaged with life.**

While these seem like things we all want, the truth is that most of us are making choices every day that actually shorten our health spans—and our life spans.

Want proof?

Well, consider this: Up to half of all premature deaths in the United States are linked to tobacco use, poor diet, and/or lack of exercise. C'mon, you're not surprised, are you?

These bad habits explain why more than half of all deaths in the United States are attributed to just three causes: heart disease, cancer, and chronic lower respiratory diseases. All of these illnesses can rob people of their health and vitality for years before they finally kill them—like a fast-forwarded aging process. And many—if not most—of these diseases can be avoided.

Knowledge Is Power

We're fortunate to be living in a time when it's easy to monitor our health and get essential information to keep ourselves well. With access to mobile apps, websites, and other health-and-wellness trackers, monitoring our numbers is easier than ever. But information helps only if you use it. And even though routine screenings and vaccinations can absolutely save lives and improve quality of life, fewer than 25 percent of people between 45 and 65 are up-to-date with their preventive care. Not good.

So set yourself up for a longer health span (and better life) by getting in the habit of health maintenance. How do you do that? It's easier than you might think: Get your health checks on schedule and talk to your doctors about whether your personal situation requires more or less frequent checkups.

Choose Wisely

There's a lot of information out there about what tests and screenings you need once you're over 45—and not all "experts" agree. While some people like to err on the side of overtesting, that approach is expensive and can result in unnecessary and even risky procedures that don't actually improve your health in the long run.

To help reduce the confusion, the American Board of Internal Medicine Foundation has partnered with a wide array of medical organizations and consumer groups, like Consumer Reports and AARP, to distribute science-based recommendations about what tests and procedures are truly the most helpful for various situations. This initiative, called Choosing Wisely, is an amazing resource to help you work with your

Telomeres: The Long and Short of Your Health Span

Take a look at your shoelaces. See those plastic caps at the ends? They're called aglets, and they're a good model for how biologists and longevity researchers picture telomeres, which are tiny protein caps on the ends of our chromosomes. Telomeres protect our chromosomes from damage, which, in turn, protects us from premature aging and many diseases. There's a direct link between the length of your telomeres and the length of your health span. Unfortunately, telomeres can be cut short by certain lifestyle factors, exposing your cells to damage and possibly an early death.

So what are these lifestyle factors? You guessed it: Stress, lack of exercise, and poor eating habits top the list. But here's some nice news: Meditation, regular exercise, and a healthy diet can actually lengthen your telomeres.

Long, healthy telomeres can correspond with a long, healthy life. So if you need one more reason to take care of yourself, think of your telomeres. Because unlike shoelaces, you can't just buy a new set.

"The most common way people give up their power is by thinking they don't have any."

—ALICE WALKER

doctors to make informed decisions about medical testing and other procedures. I've used it along with other resources to help put together the schedule below, but visit *www.choosingwisely.org* to empower yourself!

When to Do What

EVERY MONTH, DO YOUR ...

Breast self-exam. There's been a lot of discussion about breast self-exams lately, with some medical groups advising against them and others in favor. For sure, a self-exam is *never* a substitute for regular annual exams with your ob-gyn, but if you feel comfortable also doing regular checks at home, then do them right: Standing up in the shower and then again lying down, use your fingers to press all around your breasts in a circular pattern, feeling for any lumps or hard spots. Squeeze the nipple to check for any discharge. Then check in the mirror for any dimpling, puckering, or unusual changes. If anything seems out of the ordinary, call your doctor. Don't freak out—most lumps aren't cancerous. But get an expert opinion to be sure.

Skin self-exam. Using a mirror and good light, inspect your entire body closely for any new or unusual moles or skin markings. Especially be on the alert for uneven moles, new sores, or sores that don't heal, and any skin growth that looks different from what's around it. When in doubt, get it checked out by a dermatologist right away. *(See Chapter 10 for more.)*

EVERY SIX MONTHS, VISIT YOUR ...

Dentist. Visit your dentist for a dental exam and cleaning and to remove plaque and check for cavities, other gum and tooth diseases, and cancers of the mouth. *(See Chapter 8 for more.)*

EVERY ONE TO TWO YEARS, VISIT YOUR ...

Primary care physician. See your primary care physician (PCP) for a full physical exam and any recommended screenings and vaccines, and to discuss your current health and your risk for future health issues. If you have a chronic condition that requires monitoring, ask your PCP to help you set a customized schedule for more frequent checkups. And even if you're perfectly healthy right now, remember that one of the most important reasons to visit your PCP is to develop a relationship and assess your baseline health data *before* you get sick. So if you don't already have a regular doc, ask your insurance company for a list of providers and start calling.

Your PCP visits should include these tests:

• **Blood pressure test.** Get your blood pressure checked every year if you're 40 or older, and every three to five years if you're younger. If you're taking blood pressure medication or if your readings have been higher than ideal, talk to your doc about a more frequent testing schedule and consider investing in a home monitor so you can check it yourself at least once a month.

• **Basic blood work.** Your physical exam should include a blood test to evaluate your levels of white and red blood cells, as well as nutrient markers, like iron and vitamins D and B$_{12}$. This can help your PCP make sure your organs are working properly and that you aren't anemic or experiencing other nutritional deficiencies. These tests provide a baseline to help identify any changes in the future and often provide an early warning for diseases such as heart disease, diabetes, and cancer.

• **Diabetes screening.** Get your blood glucose levels checked every year or two at your physical exam. This is particularly important if you have high blood pressure, are overweight, or have other risk factors for diabetes, like a family history of the disease.

Checking In

If you're checking your blood pressure at home, you'll get the most accurate reading if you sit quietly with your feet flat on the floor and your legs uncrossed for at least 15 minutes before you take the reading. Steer clear of caffeine for a few hours prior to testing. And keep a log of your readings to discuss with your doctor.

- **Thyroid test.** TSH, the hormone produced by the thyroid gland, can fluctuate as we age, and if its levels get too high or too low, it can cause a whole slew of problems ranging from mood swings to weight gain (or loss) to cancer.

- **Electrocardiogram (EKG).** If your blood pressure and blood tests are normal, you probably don't need an EKG. However, if you have symptoms of heart disease or are at high risk, your PCP may recommend one to keep tabs on the activity of your heart and to pick up abnormal heartbeats and other cardiac issues. You may also want to consider having an EKG before starting a new exercise program if you have diabetes or another condition that can cause heart disease.

Gynecologist. Even if you're not interested in getting pregnant, you still need to visit a gynecologist regularly to screen for diseases and cancers of the reproductive organs, and to test for sexually transmitted diseases (STDs). If you're under 45 or have specific health concerns, you may need more frequent appointments. While you're there, your doc should perform the following:

- **Pelvic exam and Pap smear.** Get a pelvic exam every year and a Pap smear every three years for early detection of cervical cancer. A Pap smear screens for abnormal cells that can indicate cervical cancer, and the pelvic exam is a checkup on your reproductive organs. If you've had a hysterectomy, ask your gynecologist if—and how often—you need a Pap smear.

When Silence Isn't Golden

By the time we hit 60, at least one in three of us will have measurable hearing loss. But the condition often goes untreated for years, because it happens so gradually people don't notice until their hearing is significantly damaged. Hearing loss can lead to frustration, stress, poor memory, cognitive impairment, feelings of isolation and depression, diminished relationships and social skills—even reduced income. Treatment—typically virtually invisible hearing aids—can usually reverse these problems. But the parts of the brain that process sound can atrophy without use, so the sooner problems are addressed, the more effective treatment will be. Get tested regularly, so you can head off hearing loss before you lose out on more of life.

• **Human papillomavirus (HPV) test.** A common STD, HPV can cause genital warts and cervical cancer. Get tested with your Pap smear.

• **HIV and STD screening.** Everybody should be tested for STDs prior to engaging in sexual activity with new partners. No exceptions. Also get checked during your regular gynecological exam if you are sexually active with multiple partners or if your partner may have other partners. Some tests can be done right along with your Pap smear while others will require a separate blood test, but all should be mandatory for you and your partner.

Radiology clinic. Find yours through your PCP or ob-gyn to book a mammogram, which is used to screen for breast cancer. The American Cancer Society recommends that women age 45 to 54 get mammograms annually, while women age 55 and older can opt to switch to every two years, depending on your risk factors.

Dermatologist. Skin cancer is one of the most common cancers and is on the rise among people over 45, so get a full-body check by a dermatologist once every year—and continue to do a monthly self-check at home to look for any new or suspicious moles. If you spot one, make an appointment to get it checked out right away. A dermatologist can also help customize your skin-care routine and address any conditions with your skin or scalp. *(See Chapter 10.)*

EVERY THREE YEARS, VISIT YOUR...

Ophthalmologist. Get a baseline eye exam at age 40 to screen for glaucoma and macular degeneration and to test your vision. Then follow your ophthalmologist's recommendations—usually an exam every one to three years. *(See Chapter 9.)*

Audiologist. Get your hearing tested every 10 years until age 50, then every three years. Many PCPs can perform basic screening tests, but if yours doesn't, or if you already suspect hearing loss, see an audiologist.

EVERY FEW YEARS, CONSIDER ...

A cholesterol and triglycerides test. These types of substances can clog your arteries, and elevated levels of them often indicate heart disease. They are measured with a fasting blood test, which means that you don't eat for 9 to 12 hours before the screening. Your PCP should check your levels at least once every five years, and more often if you're diabetic or have other heart disease risk factors.

A colonoscopy. Get a colonoscopy screening starting at age 50, then every 10 years thereafter if there's no family history of colon cancer. If a parent or sibling has had colon cancer, you should get your first test 10 years before the age your relative was diagnosed. For example, if your father was diagnosed at age 57, get your first test at 47. Early detection can go a long way. Follow your PCP's orders for tests after that.

AND ASK YOUR PCP ABOUT ...

A high-sensitivity C-reactive protein (hs-CRP) test. Inflammation in the body releases hs-CRP into the bloodstream, which can be an early indicator of heart disease, type 2 diabetes, Alzheimer's disease, or other illnesses. Inflammation can have less serious causes, too, but if you're overweight and have high blood pressure or high cholesterol, or other risk factors for

Dousing the Fires of Inflammation

Inflammation has been a buzzword in medical research for a while now and has been linked to a wide range of illnesses that can shorten your life and greatly reduce your happiness. But some researchers are now looking at inflammation as a cause of aging itself. The National Institutes of Health recently made studying inflammation a top priority, but even as research continues, it seems clear that reducing inflammation throughout the body is a good idea.

So how do you lower it? For starters, get plenty of exercise and keep your weight in check. A diet loaded with fresh foods and antioxidants helps. And so does adequate rest. Visit your PCP regularly. There are some drugs that may lower hs-CRP levels—including statins—but healthy habits are an even better bet for a fire-resistant lifestyle.

Take Care of Your Bones So They Can Take Care of You

Contrary to popular belief, osteoporosis and the broken bones it can cause are not inevitable. However, reduced bone density is more likely after menopause, and the older we get the more important bone health becomes—a fractured bone can set off a domino effect of problems due to pain and lack of mobility. But the National Osteoporosis Foundation offers these simple habits to help you take charge of your bone health:

• Eat a well-balanced diet with lots of fruits and vegetables.
• Get plenty of calcium and vitamin D—including supplements if necessary.
• Do strength-training exercises regularly.
• Limit alcohol to one glass per day.
• Don't smoke.
• And if you break a bone, get a bone density test!
• Visit *www.nof.org* for all the latest information on osteoporosis.

heart disease or diabetes, discuss the test with your PCP. The ideal hs-CRP number for women is less than one milligram per liter (mg/L).

A hepatitis C test. If you were born between 1945 and 1965, consider getting this simple blood test, because hepatitis disproportionately affects your demographic—and as many as 75 percent of cases go undetected. Untreated hepatitis C can lead to liver damage, cirrhosis, and cancer, but there are effective treatments available.

A DEXA scan. DEXA is a special type of x-ray used to measure bone density. If you're over 50 and have never had one, talk with your doctor about your risk for developing osteoporosis and decide on the best time to get your first DEXA scan as a baseline for monitoring bone density in the future. And definitely talk to your doctor about getting a DEXA scan if you've fractured a bone recently.

Lung cancer screening. If you smoked—or worse, still do—then talk with your PCP about special lung cancer screenings, which may include CT scans and chest x-rays. But be aware that screenings are often inconclusive and may even result in false positives, so always get a second opinion.

Depression screening. If you feel tired, sad, and unenthusiastic about life for more than a couple of weeks, talk with your PCP about being screened for depression and finding an appropriate treatment. Depression is incredibly common, and the earlier you address it, the sooner you'll feel like yourself again.

What Vaccines Do You Need?

Vaccines are among the greatest achievements of modern medicine, and they can help you avoid not only the primary illnesses they target, but also any secondary infections or complications. Discuss this list with your PCP and get protected.

Flu vaccine. Influenza is caused by a common and highly contagious group of viruses. Most people who get the flu recover in just a week or so, but complications, including pneumonia, still kill thousands of Americans every year. For the best protection, get vaccinated annually, preferably in October or November. It's inexpensive and you can even get a flu shot at many pharmacies without an appointment. Notify your doctor's office so it can be added to your records.

Pneumonia vaccines. There are two pneumonia vaccines, given a year apart, that are recommended for people over 65 and for anyone who has a compromised immune or upper respiratory system, including people with asthma. Some people should get a booster shot after five years, but ask your PCP for a personalized time frame.

Tdap vaccine and booster. If you've never gotten the Tdap vaccine to protect against tetanus, diphtheria, and pertussis, get it now. Then get a booster (Td) shot every 10 years.

Herpes zoster (shingles) vaccine. This vaccine is strongly advised for everyone over 60, especially those who have had chicken pox. Shingles are not only painful but can lead to other problems, like hearing and vision loss, if it spreads. Luckily, vaccines can prevent the disease. There are a couple of vaccines to choose from, so talk with your PCP about the best option for you.

Taking Charge: Know Your Numbers

While age is not a measurement of health, certain numbers do offer information about your well-being. So don't just leave it up to the professionals. Pick up a simple notebook and take charge of your health by tracking the following numbers for yourself. To start, ask your PCP for a copy of the information from your most recent annual exam. And if you haven't had one recently, then you're due for a visit, aren't you?

Height. Get your height checked every year or two to make sure you're not losing inches. Some loss of height is normal as we age, but too much can indicate bone loss caused by osteoporosis or a spinal deformity like scoliosis. On average, Americans lose almost half an inch of height per decade starting at age 40, but that can be slowed by (no surprise) a healthy diet and regular exercise.

Waist size. A thickening waist isn't uncommon as we age, but it isn't inevitable and can indicate a slew of health issues, from heart disease to diabetes. So get out your tape measure and don't fudge.
Target: Under 35 inches.

Waist-to-hip ratio. Research reviewed by the Harvard School of Public Health and other organizations suggests that the proportion of your waist to your hips is also a useful predictor of heart attacks and cardiovascular disease. Measure your waist at the smallest point, then measure your hips at the widest point. Divide the first number by the second.
Target: Less than 0.85.

Blood pressure. High blood pressure, also called hypertension, is a major risk factor for heart disease and stroke. There are two blood pressure numbers that doctors measure: the systolic pressure (the higher number on top), which represents the pressure in the arteries when your heart beats, and the diastolic pressure (the lower number on the bottom), which is measured in between heartbeats.
Target: Less than 120/80.

Cholesterol level. Cholesterol is found naturally in many foods, but some cholesterol can clog arteries with plaque, increasing your risk for high blood pressure and heart disease. The American Heart Association's view on cholesterol levels has shifted over the years from a single-minded focus on numbers to a newer approach that encourages doctors to assess a patient's overall risk for heart disease

Keeping It on the Down Low

High blood pressure puts an unhealthy strain on your heart and can contribute to cardiovascular disease. So keeping your blood pressure low is important. The most critical goal is to get the systolic pressure below 120. Here are five easy ways to do just that.

INSTEAD OF EATING FAST FOODS LOADED WITH SALT,

• **Cut back on the sodium by preparing more food from scratch.** Most restaurants—especially the fast-food variety—add an enormous amount of salt, which can contribute to high blood pressure. Watch out for added salts in packaged foods from the grocery store, too.

INSTEAD OF ONE 30-MINUTE WALK EACH DAY,

• **Take three brisk 10-minute walks.** Almost any regular exercise will help, but there's strong evidence that a fast-paced 10-minute walk three times a day lowers blood pressure and helps fend off diabetes even more effectively than a single longer stroll. Even just standing up for 10 minutes out of every hour lowers blood pressure measurably.

INSTEAD OF NIBBLING ON MILK CHOCOLATE,

• **Switch to dark.** Milk chocolate has almost zero health benefits, but a square of dark chocolate every day (the kind that's at least 70 percent cacao) helps lower your blood pressure naturally. Sweet!

INSTEAD OF GUZZLING COFFEE ALL DAY,

• **Sip hibiscus tea.** While excess caffeine can raise blood pressure levels, unsweetened hibiscus tea has been demonstrated to lower blood pressure as much as 7 percent in people with prehypertensive levels. Drink three or more cups daily to help naturally—and deliciously—lower blood pressure. Try it iced, too.

INSTEAD OF GIVING UP IF THOSE NUMBERS WON'T BUDGE,

• **Ask your doctor about medications.** No matter how healthy your lifestyle, you may have a genetic predisposition for high blood pressure. In that case, medication might be the extra boost you need—but keep making good choices, too, so you can keep your dose as low as possible to reduce side effects.

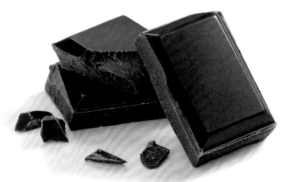

and stroke, and consider the ratio between HDL ("good" cholesterol) and LDL ("bad"), as well as total levels.

Target: A total under 200 milligrams per deciliter (mg/dL), with HDL above 60 and LDL under 60.

Triglycerides level. Triglycerides are another substance found in your blood, and another indicator of potential cardiovascular disease. The American Heart Association says a level under 150 is acceptable for most women. Get triglycerides checked along with cholesterol, and discuss the results with your doctor.

Target: 150 mg/dL is normal, 100 mg/dL is optimal.

Blood sugar (glucose) level. Blood sugar levels normally fluctuate during the course of the day, but your ability to regulate them can decrease as you age, potentially leading to diabetes. The most effective ways to regulate blood sugar are exercising every day and cutting back on simple carbohydrates, like sugar. If you've been diagnosed with diabetes, your doc may suggest you start tracking your blood sugar at home with a glucose meter.

Target: Under 100 mg/dL.

Vitamin D level. Most of us know vitamin D is important for helping with the absorption of calcium and reducing the risk of osteoporosis, but there's evidence it can reduce the risk of other diseases as well. Our bodies can make vitamin D from sunlight, but not all of us get enough, so your levels should be checked as part of your regular blood work.

Target: Typically 30 to 50 nanograms per milliliter (ng/mL) or higher, but vitamin D needs vary depending on factors like race, age, weight, and lifestyle, so talk to your PCP about your specific needs.

Taking the Pulse of Heart Health

According to the American Heart Association, the resting heart rate for most healthy women is between 60 and 100 beats per minute. However, a Women's Health Initiative study found that women who had resting heart rates of more than 76 beats per minute were 26 percent more likely to have a heart attack than those whose heart rates were close to 60.

Best time to check your resting heart rate? First thing in the morning, before you get out of bed.

The best way to get it down to 60? You guessed it: Exercise!

Resting heart rate. Your pulse, especially measured while you're sitting still, is a key indicator of cardiovascular health, so check your heart rate regularly. Here's how: Put two fingers on your pulse—either at your neck or wrist—and count how many beats you feel in 15 seconds. Multiply that number by four to get beats per minute. Or you can do what I do and wear a fitness band to monitor your pulse continuously—even while sleeping.
Target: Between 60 and 100 beats per minute, but closer to 60 is best.

Beyond the Baseline

Okay, so we've taken the first steps toward monitoring our health. But how can we use that information to *stay* healthy? Easy. By regarding these numbers as a starting point, doing whatever we need to do to move them closer to our targets, tracking them (regularly, and in writing!) so we're alert to any changes, and seeking professional help to address problems early before they have a chance to do serious damage. These simple actions will go a long way toward helping our bodies work as well as possible for as long as possible.

Know Your Risk

It's true that, on average, women tend to stay healthier longer than men. But as we age, some problems actually affect us more often. These common ailments aren't necessarily the biggest killers of women—those would be heart disease and cancer—but they can significantly impact your ability to enjoy life and can raise your risk of more serious problems down the road.

Autoimmune disease. This isn't one illness but a whole category of diseases in which the immune system mistakenly attacks other body parts and systems. Most autoimmune disorders are chronic, and several—including Graves' disease, multiple sclerosis, lupus, and rheumatoid arthritis—disproportionately affect women. Diagnosis may take time and may include physical exams as well as blood and imaging tests.
Watch for: Ongoing fatigue, pain, dizziness, swelling, fever, abdominal cramps, rashes, or other persistent symptoms that can't be explained. Seek treatment early; these diseases can increase inflammation in the body, creating a higher risk for heart disease.
Risk factors: Genetics or exposure to certain toxins, like industrial solvents and heavy metals, are linked to some autoimmune disorders, but some other autoimmune issues are harder to explain.

Have You Checked In With Your Chi Today?

When I recently suffered a herniated disc, my doctor sent me to a practitioner of traditional Chinese medicine (TCM). TCM, which has been practiced in the East for more than 2,500 years, uses a combination of acupuncture, diet, and special herbs to improve the way the whole body functions, rather than just treating individual symptoms. TCM practitioners spend an hour or more examining each patient and asking questions about health and lifestyle before developing customized treatments. The goal is to maximize health throughout the body by focusing on the relationships between diet, exercise, lifestyle, stress, and overall wellness.

ACUPUNCTURE TO THE RESCUE

While Western science is still studying the efficacy of traditional Chinese herbs and other aspects of TCM, the use of acupuncture was recognized by the National Institutes of Health back in 1997 as a viable treatment option for certain conditions. Acupuncture is a method of stimulating the body's natural healing systems by placing thin needles into the skin at strategic points. While it sounds painful, the needles create only a small twinge when they are inserted. After all the needles are in place, you simply rest and relax for at least 15 minutes. Acupuncture has been shown to effectively reduce back and neck problems, chronic pain, nausea, migraines, acute injuries, respiratory and neurological disorders, and more.

As for me, I can happily report that it totally resolved the pain from my herniated disc.

PREVENTION BEFORE CURE

In addition to giving us acupuncture, TCM has another important lesson to offer us Westerners: Our focus should be on *maintaining* health, rather than fixing problems after the fact.

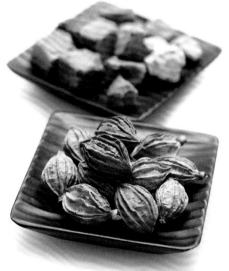

Andrew Weil, director of the Center for Integrative Medicine at the University of Arizona, and arguably America's best known advocate of an integrated approach to wellness, believes that TCM's emphasis on prevention is an idea we all need to embrace, whether through TCM or Western preventive care, if we are to truly live our best lives as we get older.

Chronic fatigue syndrome (CFS). This little-understood disorder causes debilitating fatigue and muscle pain, but because there are no external symptoms and no clear cause, CFS has been controversial among physicians and researchers trying to diagnose and treat it. Women suffer from CFS four times more often than men.

Watch for: Extreme fatigue that does not improve with sleep, joint pain with no swelling, and loss of memory and concentration.

Risk factors: Largely unknown, but chronic stress may increase your risk.

Depression. Women are almost twice as likely to suffer from depression as men as we age. This may be due to a combination of factors, including hormonal changes and longer life expectancy, which can lead to loneliness.

Watch for: Prolonged feelings (more than two weeks) of sadness or hopelessness, fatigue, persistent negative thoughts, and loss of interest in activities that you used to enjoy.

Risk factors: Depression can affect anyone, but risk goes up with big life changes, like divorce or retirement, an increase in isolation, inadequate exercise, and underlying health conditions.

Gallstones. By the time they reach 75, as many as half of all women will develop gallstones—tiny hard particles that get trapped in the gallbladder. If caught early, gallstones are easy to treat, but left untreated, they can cause painful and serious complications.

Watch for: Sudden and intense abdominal pain.

Risk factors: Genetics, having diabetes, taking birth control pills or hormone therapy, being overweight, undergoing rapid weight loss, and eating a diet high in carbohydrates and low in fiber.

Hypertension (aka high blood pressure). According to the U.S. Centers for Disease Control and Prevention (CDC), heart disease is the #1 killer of women in the United States, and high blood pressure is a major risk factor. Kidney disease—a major contributor to hypertension—also affects women more often than men and is a big risk factor.

Watch for: There are few symptoms of high blood pressure, which is why it's called the silent killer, so it's best to get your blood pressure checked regularly.

Risk factors: Genetics, having diabetes, eating too much salt, getting too little exercise, and being overweight.

Irritable bowel syndrome (IBS). IBS is a common disorder that causes severe bloating and pain in the large intestine, and may affect up to 10 to 15 percent of Americans at some point in their lives.

Watch for: Bloating, abdominal pain, constipation, and/or diarrhea.

Risk factors: Largely unknown. Risk may increase with food allergies, hormonal fluctuations, and stress.

Migraines. Many more women than men suffer from debilitating migraines—often throughout their lives—until they go through menopause. Once estrogen takes a nosedive, migraines seem to settle down, too.

Watch for: Severe headaches, possibly accompanied by an upset stomach and vision problems.

Risk factors: Stress, caffeine, alcohol, salty foods, hormonal fluctuations, medications like birth control pills, and vasodilators like nitroglycerin.

Osteoporosis. Osteoporosis is the primary reason that half of all women over 50 will fracture a bone, compared with one in four men. The biggest reason for loss of bone mass is the drop in estrogen that occurs with menopause, but diet and exercise can affect bone density as well.

Watch for: There are few early symptoms, but over time, osteoporosis may contribute to loss of height. Monitor bone density with periodic DEXA scans.

Risk factors: Genetics, age, other medical conditions, certain medications, lack of exercise, poor diet, and low levels of vitamin D.

Stroke. Stroke is the third most common cause of death for American women, but fast treatment has been proven to save lives and greatly reduce long-term damage. Many women experience short mini-strokes, called transient ischemic attacks (TIAs), starting months or years before a full stroke. Treating TIAs quickly can reduce the risk of stroke later in life.

Watch for: Sudden onset of numbness or weakness—especially on one side of the face or body, sudden confusion, sudden slurring of speech, and sudden headache or dizziness. The big clue is "sudden," so if you have any of these symptoms, call 911 immediately.

Risk factors: High blood pressure, smoking, heart disease, diabetes, taking birth control pills or hormone replacement therapy, and having TIAs.

Thyroid disease. As we age, women are at a higher risk for thyroid disorders, in which our glands start producing either too much or too little of the thyroid hormones. Too little hormone production is called hypothyroid-ism, while too much is hyperthyroidism. Both are difficult to diagnose and are often confused with other conditions, which is why getting your thyroid levels checked regularly is essential so any changes are easy to spot.

Watch for: Unexplained fluctuations in weight or energy levels; mood swings.

Risk factors: Genetics and age; thyroid disease is most common after 60.

Urinary tract problems. Women are more likely to contract urinary tract infections (UTIs) and experience incontinence than men.

Watch for: Pain while urinating, the urge to urinate suddenly or frequently, pain in the lower abdomen, and leaking urine accidentally.

Risk factors for UTIs: Diabetes, using diaphragms, and hormone changes.

Risk factors for incontinence: Age, having diabetes, past pregnancies, being overweight, and loss of muscle tone in pelvis.

These are just some of the health issues we may encounter as we age, so always be vigilant about how you're feeling, and discuss any sudden changes or persistent symptoms with your doctor. And if your body is screaming out for attention, listen to it! Cross my healthy heart, I won't call you a hypochondriac.

10 Small Steps to a Longer Health Span

❶ Keep track of your health numbers, especially height, waist size, resting heart rate, and blood pressure.

❷ Take care of your bones with diet and daily strength training.

❸ Do breast and skin self-exams every month—and get a second opinion immediately if something seems off.

❹ See your dentist every six months.

❺ See your PCP, gynecologist, and dermatologist every one to two years for checkups and screenings.

❻ See an ophthalmologist every one to three years for a vision check and glaucoma test.

❼ See an audiologist for a hearing test every 10 years until age 50, then every three years.

❽ Get vaccines on schedule.

❾ Follow Choosing Wisely guidelines for medical exams and tests.

❿ Focus on prevention first, but pay attention to your body, and seek help ASAP if anything seems amiss.

A Healthier You

If you want to look and feel great for as long as you live—and maybe even make your life itself longer—here's a prescription for healthy habits:

INSTEAD OF VIEWING EXERCISE AS AN OCCASIONAL CHORE,
Move your body every single day.
(See Chapter 2.)

INSTEAD OF EATING WHATEVER'S FAST AND CHEAP,
Give your body the quality fuel it needs to be strong and healthy.
(See Chapter 3.)

INSTEAD OF STAYING UP HALF THE NIGHT TO WATCH TV
OR SCROLL THROUGH INSTAGRAM,
Get enough sleep for the stamina to live a full life. *(See Chapter 4.)*

INSTEAD OF BASKING IN THE SUN OR, WORSE, BAKING IN A TANNING BED,
Wear sunscreen and sun-protective clothing to keep your skin safe from UV rays.
(See Chapter 10.)

INSTEAD OF KNOCKING BACK HALF A BOTTLE OF WINE EACH NIGHT,
Limit alcohol to one drink a day.

INSTEAD OF ASSUMING EITHER THAT YOU'RE INVINCIBLE
OR THAT ILLNESS IS INEVITABLE,
Get real and get your exams, screenings, and vaccines as needed. You might even schedule them around your birthday, as an annual gift to yourself.

INSTEAD OF TRYING TO REMEMBER WHICH VACCINES TO GET WHEN,
Ask your doctor's office to alert you with a reminder call, email, or postcard—and then book your appointment right away.

INSTEAD OF LYING TO YOUR DOCTOR BECAUSE
YOU'RE CONCERNED SHE MIGHT JUDGE YOU,
Be honest and open with physicians so they can understand what's going on, diagnose any problems accurately, and help you take care of yourself.

INSTEAD OF ONLY TREATING SYMPTOMS,
Find the root problem and fix it. Pain pills, sleeping aids, and other medications can give you short-term relief when something goes wrong, but if you keep using them without addressing the underlying health issue, you're setting yourself up for long-term unhappiness. Aim for maximum health, not a minimum quick fix.

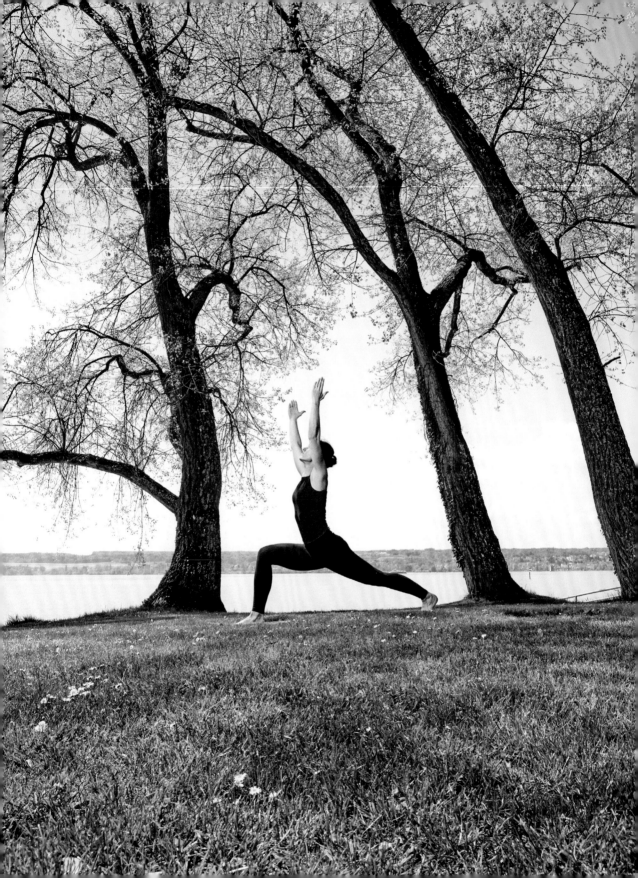

CHAPTER 2

All Roads Lead to Fitness

"Physical fitness is not only one of the most important keys to a healthy body; it is the basis of dynamic and creative intellectual activity."

—JOHN F. KENNEDY

Feeling sluggish, gaining weight, or not sleeping well? Think that being tired, grumpy, lumpy, and stressed is what getting older is all about?

Sure, you'd like to take better care of yourself, you say, but there are so many other things to worry about: your kids, spouse, parents, jobs, communities, friends. The list is endless, right? I know that list all too well.

I also know how convincing the flow of excuses seems, until even you believe you can't possibly make a change: *No time. Can't do it. Too busy. Too stressed. Too tired.*

But if you really want to take good care of your kids, parents, and jobs; if you want to improve your mood and have more energy; if you want to reduce that stress; if you want to keep your brain sharp, bones strong, and immune system solid; and if you want to live a vital, vibrant, and longer life, here's my best advice:

Get more exercise.

Wait! Stay with me! I know you're sick of hearing about what's supposedly wrong with your physique and how everything needs improving. I sure am. Just walk past any newsstand and you'll be slapped in the face with a bunch of taut, supple (and heavily photoshopped) young bodies next to headlines that order us to flatten those abs, sculpt that butt, and lose 10 pounds. It's as if they want us to be ashamed of ... what? Being over 25? Don't fall for it!

"*Fitness—if it came in a bottle, everybody would have a great body.*"

—CHER

The truth is, no matter how far past 25 you are, adding exercise into your daily or weekly routine is pretty much the best guarantee of a quality life that you can give yourself. And it's easier than you might think. Seriously! It's just about (wait for it!) taking small steps to get more fit. And the fitter you are, the more energy you'll have to take the next steps. And, yes, you'll also feel—and look—younger. But most important, you'll fit more living into your life.

How to Take Back Your Body, One Step at a Time

The list of benefits you'll reap from regular exercise is nearly endless. But if your will to get started is flagging, or other tasks still seem more important, just remember:

Exercise will make you feel good almost immediately.

Even moderate levels of exertion, such as walking, will trigger your nervous system to increase the production of endorphins, which make you feel more alert and energized. Endorphins are the body's natural opioids, and intense exercise produces enough of them to create what's known as a runner's high. But that's not all. Exercise can also quickly suppress production of cortisol, the stress hormone, and increase happiness hormones, like serotonin and dopamine. Result? A better mood, improved critical thinking skills, and less anxiety during your workout and for hours afterward.

True or False?

EXERCISING CAN BRING ON AN ORGASM.

True. This phenomenon is nicknamed "coregasm," according to human sexuality professor Debra Herbenick, who says that about 10 percent of women and men have experienced it. Coregasms don't have to involve friction on your genitals or any thoughts about sex at all. They usually result from extended squeezing of the abdominal, pelvic, and leg muscles. So how about doing another set of those hanging leg lifts?

How Hard and How Much?

Those are the big questions, right? The short answer is that more is always better. But that's not the whole story. For the best cardiovascular health, the American Heart Association recommends a minimum of:

Thirty minutes of moderate aerobic activity five days a week, for a total of 150 minutes per week, *or* **25 minutes of vigorous aerobic activity** three days a week, for a total of 75 minutes per week, *plus* **muscle-strengthening activity** at least two days a week.

But remember, these are minimums. As long as you don't overwork yourself to the point of injury, do as much as you can. Some research suggests that the most important factor may actually be the frequency of activity—so if you tend to sit for hours at a stretch, make a point of getting up more often.

HOW TO GAUGE INTENSITY

• Moderate aerobic activity means you're sweating a little after 10 minutes and you're breathing harder than normal but you can still carry on a conversation. Your heart rate will be between 50 and 75 percent of maximum.

• Vigorous aerobic activity means you're sweating after a few minutes and your breaths are deep and rapid. You can talk but have to pause often to catch your breath. Your heart rate will be between 70 and 85 percent of maximum.

MAXIMUM HEART RATE

Maximum heart rate—how many times your heart can beat per minute—will vary according to your body type and fitness level. For a rough measure, subtract your age from 220—if you're 50, your maximum heart rate will be about 170 beats per minute. Therefore, moderate activity should put you at 85 to 119 beats per minute, while vigorous activity should put you between 119 and 145 beats.

Optimal aerobic benefits come at about 75 percent of maximum heart rate, but even gentle exercise will help increase your fitness level and reduce your health risks.

When you're just beginning a new exercise program, aim to peak at about 50 percent of your maximum heart rate during your first few weeks, then gradually increase intensity until your workouts peak close to 80 percent of maximum—but *never* go over that 85 percent mark.

Nag Alert! Here's What Happens When You Don't Move Your Body

- According to data from the CDC, approximately 36 percent of adults in the United States do not engage in any leisure-time physical activity. This lack of activity, according to a study published in the *American Journal of Medicine,* contributes to 22 percent of coronary heart disease diagnoses, 22 percent of colon cancers, and 18 percent of osteoporotic fractures, among other problems.
- A report in the medical journal the *Lancet* estimated that lack of physical activity is responsible for as many as one in 10 premature deaths worldwide.
- For women over 30, physical inactivity may be the single greatest contributor to the risk of heart disease. Among women age 22 to 27, it's smoking.
- A Brazilian study found that people between the ages of 51 and 80 who needed to use their hands and knees to sit down on the floor and stand back up were almost seven times more likely to die within six years, compared with those who could get up and down without support. Yikes!
- Lack of exercise can exacerbate anxiety and depression.
- Not moving costs money! A study published in the *Lancet* calculated that not exercising costs the world almost $68 billion a year in medical expenses and lost productivity due to diseases directly tied to inactivity. A different study, published in the *Journal of the American Heart Association*, estimated that Americans who already have cardiovascular disease will save an average of $2,500 a year in health care expenses just by meeting weekly exercise guidelines.

ON THE OTHER HAND: HERE'S WHAT HAPPENS WHEN YOU DO MOVE EVERY DAY

- Researchers from the University of California, San Francisco and the University of Mississippi found that people who exercise regularly show fewer signs of aging in their cells. Intriguingly, the correlation is strongest for people between 40 and 64, which suggests that midlife is a critical time to gain the long-term benefits of exercise. These benefits also appear to be directly linked to the amount and variety of exercise that study participants took part in. The bottom line: More exercise means younger, healthier cells.

• A study published in the *European Heart Journal* showed that being "metabolically fit"—which researchers said was largely influenced by exercise—reduces a person's chances of dying prematurely by 38 percent, even if he or she is considerably overweight.

• Regular exercise helps keep blood pressure low, muscles toned, bones dense, and sleep deep. It has also been shown to reduce stress, mild anxiety, and mild depression.

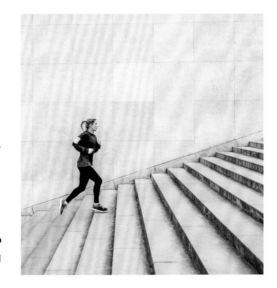

• Research conducted on Senior Olympians calculated that the older athletes' average fitness age is 20 or more years younger than their chronological age. And while you can't change your chronological age, you can absolutely change your fitness age—through increased exercise.

• Researchers at the University of Texas Southwestern Medical Center and the Cooper Institute in Dallas found that the speed at which we can run a mile has a direct correlation with our overall fitness and risk of developing heart disease. For a woman in her 50s, a nine-minute mile is considered high fitness and only an 11.9 percent lifetime chance of heart problems. If a woman of the same age takes 12 or more minutes to run a mile, she has low fitness and a 27.8 percent chance of heart disease. The good news? You can always improve your fitness!

TO SUMMARIZE:

• Want to fight or fix heart disease? Exercise.
• Need to lose or maintain weight? Exercise.
• Determined to ditch the stress? Exercise.
• Aim to ax your risk factors for certain cancers? Exercise.
• Trying to dodge diabetes? Exercise.
• Focused on keeping blood pressure low? Exercise.
• Thinking of your telomeres? Exercise

Exercise will help you sleep better, be stronger, and dramatically increase your chances of living a vibrant life as you age. And, hey, it'll make those new jeans look better, too.

Moving your body increases blood circulation, which means more oxygen going not only to your muscles but also to your brain, boosting concentration and memory. That's why taking a 10-minute walk break in the afternoon can actually make you more productive than sitting at your desk for another hour. And you'll sleep better, too, which means you'll be more alert and effective tomorrow.

I jump-started my own journey back to feeling great simply by increasing my physical activity. And there is nothing unique about my story. All bodies—no matter the specific challenges that each body has—work better when we make them work.

Step 1: Move your body. Every day.

If you take nothing else from this book, please take this: The most important thing you can do for yourself, from your brain to your heart to your skin to your peace of mind, is to move. Play tennis or basketball, dance, swim, hike, ride a bike, or do Zumba. Gardening counts, as does strenuous housecleaning, or even carrying heavy bags of groceries. If you have physical challenges or handicaps, there are adaptive sports organizations all across the country to help you find your active passion. Whatever you do, choose something that gets your heart beating and body moving for at least 30 to 60 minutes every day. And duration matters less than frequency: You'll still benefit from regular movement even if you break it up into short sessions throughout the day. So check with your doc to make sure you don't have preexisting conditions that might be aggravated by your preferred activities—then get active!

Step 2: Take a hike.

The next step, literally, is to walk more. Or run, if you prefer. Work yourself up to 10,000 steps a day if you can, but any little bit will help. A simple pedometer or fitness tracker will help keep you on target. Every step counts, whether it's through a mall, up a hill, or running toward a soccer goal. Take a long walk—or several short ones. If you need an extra push to get outside, adopt a dog (mine's named Gunther). Whatever it takes to get you going, just do it.

Walking is pretty much the perfect exercise. Think about it:

It's easy, free, requires no special equipment (although comfortable shoes do help), and you can do it anywhere, anytime.

Need more convincing? A study released in 2015 by the London School of Economics found that people who walked at a brisk pace for at least 30 minutes several times a week had smaller waist circumferences and lower body mass indices (BMIs) than people who spent the same amount of time doing moderate-intensity sports like swimming and cycling, gym-based exercises, or other moderate-intensity activities. And what defines a brisk pace? Anything fast enough to increase your heart rate will do.

Tip: Fit an extra step in. When you must drive, park at the far side of the lot so you can get more steps on your pedometer. At the grocery store, take your cart back to the store entrance when you're done. It's good exercise *and* good manners!

The Fastest Burn at the Gym

According to data from Harvard, pedaling a stationary bike or using a ski machine provides the fastest calorie burns of all gym equipment activities—391 calories during a vigorous 30-minute stationary bike workout and 353 calories for 30 minutes of skiing for a 155-pound person.

Step 3: Get strong (because that's the new sexy).

For firm arms, strong bones, and a taut tush, as well as overall toning and health, strength training should be a critical part of your wellness routine. It's just as important as your cardio exercises. For targeted results, I asked multiple fitness experts for their best-of-the-best recommendations, but remember: These should be combined with cardio and balance activities for full fitness. For maximum results, complete each exercise at least five times a week. But that won't be hard, because these exercises don't take long and will fit easily into your day.

THE THREE BEST EXERCISES TO PROTECT YOUR BONES

Running. It's a cardio staple, but it's also a weight-bearing exercise, which makes it great for bone density, too. And it's never too late to start. I was nearly 50 when I first began running, and I haven't stopped yet!

Jumping. Frog leaps, jumping jacks, and jump-roping are all great options. They'll boost your cardio, sure, but they'll also do wonders for your leg bones and hips. *Bonus:* You don't need much room to practice them. Or try burpees for a full-body strength workout.

Push-ups. A fantastic exercise for oh-so-many reasons. Push-ups strengthen your core and tone your arms, which helps you look and feel great but also means you can catch yourself safely if you ever fall. Push-ups also put weight on your arm bones and shoulders, which helps keep them strong. Aim to do 12 to 20 push-ups per day.

THE THREE BEST EXERCISES FOR A GREAT REAR VIEW

A firm derrière certainly makes you feel sexy, but strong glutes also help you walk, run, and stand straight and tall—especially as you age.

Plié squats. Stand with your legs spread a little more than shoulder width apart and your feet turned out. Slowly squat down, pushing your butt as far back as you can (this helps protect your knees). Hold for a few seconds, then slowly squeeze your muscles to stand back up. Repeat 20 times.

Planks. The plank works your entire body, including the core. Here's how to do it: Get into alignment for your preferred push-up, extend your arms—and hold it. That's it! Keep your abs pulled in and your hips level with your shoulders. Start by holding the plank for short periods a few times a day, and work up to 30 seconds at a time ... then 45 ... then 60, up to two minutes. If that gets too easy, hold for even longer or alternate lifting one leg at a time. If the regular plank bothers your wrists, try doing it on your fists (knuckles down) or do a forearm plank by placing your forearms on the ground with your elbows under your shoulders and your hands turned out slightly to the sides.

Take That Coffee Break

Several recent studies suggest that caffeine can boost your workout by improving circulation, easing post-workout recovery, increasing calorie burn, and reducing the risk of age-related injuries. Consuming 12 to 16 ounces of coffee or black tea an hour before a workout seems to give the best effects. But timing matters: If caffeine comes less than six hours before bedtime, it could affect your sleep, which would negate these benefits.

For Full Fitness, You Need Three Key Ingredients

Just moving more—in any way—is going to improve your well-being, no question. But if you want to maximize your fitness and health, then give your body the three different kinds of conditioning it needs for the long haul.

AEROBIC CONDITIONING will improve your lung capacity and strengthen your cardio-vascular system, which in turn will increase your daily energy and stamina, and reduce your risk of heart disease, diabetes, and other ailments. It will also help you burn fat and maintain a healthy weight.
• TIP: You get aerobic benefits from anything that raises your heart rate and gets you breathing more heavily. Try walking, running, biking, or swimming (and sex counts!). If you've implemented Steps 1 and 2, you're already there.

STRENGTH BUILDING is critical for preserving bone strength and density as well as for toning muscles. We can start to lose bone mass as we approach menopause, or even earlier. However, according to the National Osteoporosis Foundation, a regular regimen of weight-bearing and muscle-strengthening exercises can help maintain bone density and protect against osteoporosis. Any activity that forces your body to work against gravity or resistance counts. In addition, strong abdominal and back muscles—aka your "core"—help maintain good posture and protect against back injuries and falls.
• TIP: Non-weight-bearing exercises, like swimming and cycling, can be great for cardio and muscle-toning but do little to fight osteoporosis, so if those are your primary fit-ness activities, you'll need to incorporate targeted weight-bearing exercises, too. *(See Step 3.)*

BALANCE AND FLEXIBILITY tend to decline gradually as we age, and the resulting falls and accidents often kick off a downward spiral of problems. However, you can preserve and even regain balance and flexibility through regular (read: daily) practice. Ordinary stretching helps, as does any activity that forces you to bend and shift your body, like dancing, yoga, Pilates, rock climbing, and martial arts.
• TIP: Improve your balance throughout your day by lifting one foot at a time off the ground when you're waiting in line, doing dishes, or watching TV.

Use Your Smartphone to Get Health-Smart

When I go for a run, I take my phone with me. Sure, it's good for emergencies, but I also use it to listen to Tom Petty and the Heartbreakers, which keeps my pace up and my brain cells percolating. If I spot a hawk circling above Central Park, I can snap a photo, which makes me happy, and in turn healthier. What's more, I can text the photo to my husband and daughters, which boosts our relationships. Pretty cool, right? That little gadget is packed with health-improving tools, including apps that help you reach your wellness goals:

Track your progress. While I still love my fitness wristband, I don't really need it now that smartphones come with sensors to measure steps taken, calories burned, and more. Most have a preloaded health app that can activate all these functions, so check the specs on your model. For those of us who prefer wearable trackers, we can download the data right to our phones and easily monitor our progress and habits on our screens.

Track your workouts. And plan them, too! There are several apps available that guide you through workouts with coaching tips, instructional videos, and a workout log. One of the most popular is the Nike+ Training Club app, but there are new ones popping up all the time.

Track your runs and rides. If you're a competitive runner or cyclist, try Strava to record your times and distances and to motivate yourself by "racing" against other users. If you prefer a different kind of motivation, Charity Miles is a free app that gets corporations to donate a few cents to a charity of your choice for every mile that you walk, run, or bike. Win-win!

Track your meals. MyFitnessPal is one of many apps that offer a calorie counter, as well as add-ons for even more diet and exercise info. Use it to track what you eat.

Track your heart rate. Your phone can help you monitor your resting heart rate anytime by turning the camera into a heart rate sensor. There are several good apps available, including Instant Heart Rate and Fit Heart.

Track your sleep. Your phone can check on sleep patterns, too. Try Sleep Cycle, which uses your phone's microphone to analyze your movements during sleep, allowing it to track your sleep patterns and even wake you gently at the optimal time.

All this and it makes calls, too.

Wall squats. Stand with your feet hip-width apart a few inches from a wall. With your back flat against the wall, slowly lower yourself to a sitting position, with your knees bent at a 90-degree angle, and hold for 10 to 30 seconds, depending on your ability. Come back up to standing for 20 to 30 seconds. Repeat 20 times.

THREE EXERCISES FOR POWERFUL ARMS

One of the first things I noticed when I reached my 40s was how weak my arms were getting. The good news is that a few simple (but challenging) exercises can gain that strength back—and more. The better news is we're already practicing two out of three.

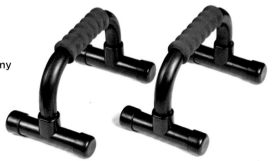

A Very Proper Push-Up

The push-up is a powerful exercise that strengthens several parts of your body. However, it's important to do it right, because improper form can create too much stress on your wrists, back, and shoulders. Try one of these techniques:

• **Full push-ups.** Start on your hands and knees, placing your hands under your shoulders, with your fingers facing slightly outward. Step your feet back and straighten your legs until your body is in a long, firm line, with your back straight. Holding your abs in and keeping your legs strong, bend your elbows— hugging them in toward your ribs—until your upper arms are parallel with the floor. Stay steady and keep breathing as you slowly push yourself back up.

• **Modified push-ups.** If the full deal is too much at first (and it is for most of us), start out by keeping your knees on the floor. If that's still too intense, then work on standing push-ups by placing your hands on a wall and your feet a foot or two away. Stick with your preferred modification or gradually work your way into a full push-up.

Whatever version you choose to do, move slowly and deliberately, keeping good alignment with a strong core and elbows close to your ribs. Lower your body on a count of eight, hold this position for eight, and then take eight counts on the way back up. And remember: It's better to do fewer strong push-ups than more sloppy ones. And keep practicing!

Push-ups. Check!

Planks. Check!

Backward chair push-ups. Grab a sturdy chair and put it behind you. Bend your knees until you can place your hands on the front edge of the seat. Cross your legs. Keep your back straight as you slowly lower yourself down as far as you can go, then slowly push back up. Work up to 20 repetitions.

Putting It All Together

Are you ready to kick-start your fitness habit? Here's your action plan:

❶ Get measured.

Make sure you have a handle on your health-check numbers from Chapter 1. Not only will they alert you to any health issues you need to focus on, but they'll give you a baseline you can use to compare your progress, which can be very motivating!

❷ Get the green light.

If you have any preexisting health issues or haven't been active in a while, check in with your PCP to get the go-ahead before making any big changes in your diet or

For These Women, Age Is Just a Number

• **Diana Nyad** was 64 years old when she became the first person to swim the 110 miles from Havana, Cuba, to Key West, Florida, without a shark cage.

• **Ernestine Shepherd** started competing in bodybuilding competitions in 1992 at the ripe young age of 56. She has since won two bodybuilding titles and participated in nine marathons.

• **Harriette Thompson** became the oldest woman to run a marathon when she finished the 2015 Rock 'n' Roll San Diego Marathon at the age of 92.

• **Sister Madonna Buder** was 48 when she first took up jogging. The "Iron Nun" has since completed over 340 triathlons. In 2012 she set a world record for oldest Ironman finisher—at age 82.

exercise routine. Of course, that will be easy, since you'll already be at the doctor's office to get your health-check tests, right?

❸ Get equipped.

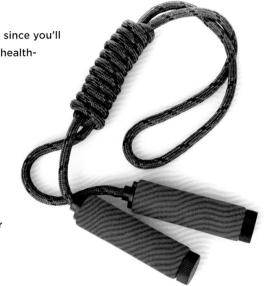

I strongly recommend a simple pedometer or fitness tracker to count your daily steps. You can also use your phone to track your progress. Otherwise, all you really need are some comfortable clothes and a good pair of running shoes—or whatever suits your favorite activity.

❹ Get going!

No matter how old you are, you—yes, you—can change your body, your fitness level, how you feel, and how good the rest of your life is going to be. Just moving more will be the one habit that makes the biggest difference in your life. It won't take a miracle, but it will take a commitment to make yourself your first priority.

10 Small Steps to a Lifelong Fitness Habit

❶ Stand as often as possible.

❷ Incorporate as much movement into your life as you can.

❸ Walk as much as you can, aiming for 10,000 or more steps every day.

❹ Exercise for at least 30 minutes, five times a week; or crank out vigorous exercise for 25 minutes, three times a week.

❺ For maximum health, include cardio, strength building, and balance exercises several times a week.

❻ Get your heart rate up to at least 50 percent of your maximum for a minimum of 15 minutes every time you exercise.

❼ Do push-ups, planks, plié squats, wall squats, and chair dips as many days as possible.

❽ Find activities that make you happy while you're doing them.

❾ Set goals that get you excited.

❿ Don't give up!

Your Best Bod

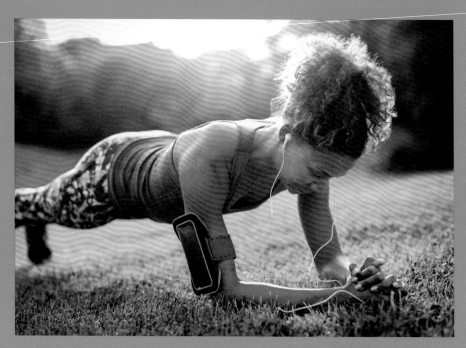

Here are some tried-and-true strategies to keep you on the path of fitness for life.

INSTEAD OF THINKING OF EXERCISE AS A CHORE,

Do what you love. You're more likely to do things that give you immediate rewards—like a better mood and less stress. So pick activities that you truly enjoy, mixing it up during each day or week to include cardio, strength, and balance.

INSTEAD OF GIVING UP AFTER TWO WEEKS,

Give it three months. Research shows most life changes take three months to become habit. This was certainly true for me. When I first started getting in shape a few years ago, I pledged to stick with my new routine—running three times a week for three months. Sure enough, in that time I saw my health, fitness, and life turn around so much that I celebrated my 50th birthday by running my first marathon!

INSTEAD OF EXERCISING FOR THE SAKE OF EXERCISING,

Set a goal. No, not a weight-loss goal. Keep your motivation strong by setting a new personal challenge every month or two, like running a local 5K. You'll be even more likely to stick to your training if you make your goal public, so tell everyone what you're doing—and post updates on social media to share your enthusiasm.

INSTEAD OF GOING IT ALONE,

Make it social. Find a fitness buddy (or two) and turn your workouts into a social outing. If you can't always exercise together, use a pedometer or fitness app to compare progress and set group goals—or start a healthy competition! Or seek out a club, or search websites like *Meetup.com* to locate like-minded fitness partners.

INSTEAD OF REARRANGING YOUR SCHEDULE AROUND YOUR WORKOUTS,

Fit your workouts into your schedule. You don't have to get all of your exercise in one dose. In fact, some studies show it may be healthier to spread your exercise throughout the day. Go for a run before work and do some yoga in the afternoon, then round up the whole family for a bike ride after dinner.

INSTEAD OF LETTING FITNESS SLIDE WHEN YOU GET BUSY,

Commit to yourself. Treat your exercise plans like every other important appointment. Put them in your calendar and show up on time—even if it's a solo workout.

INSTEAD OF SITTING ALL DAY,

Create walk breaks. Set an alarm to remind you to get up every 20 minutes and walk around, even if it's just down the hall of your office or around your living room. Put your laptop on a counter and check your email or read the news standing up.

INSTEAD OF GOING TO THE GYM,

Bring the gym home. You can do a whole workout without leaving the house! *For cardio:* Do jumping jacks, run in place, and run up and down a staircase, for 60 seconds each. Repeat the circuit five or six times. *For strength training:* Do 20 push-ups, 20 plié squats, and 20 backward chair push-ups, and hold a plank for 60 seconds. Repeat the circuit three times. *To cool down:* Walk around your home until your heart rate slows to near normal. Lie on the floor, hug your knees to your chest, and roll back and forth. Finish with a few gentle stretches and hit the shower, champ!

INSTEAD OF GETTING BORED,

Shake it up. Find a variety of activities you love and keep them in rotation, whether you change daily or seasonally. And don't be afraid to try new things. If you run, try biking once a week. Take up swimming for the summer, or go stand-up paddle-boarding or rowing. If you walk or run on a treadmill, head outside on sunny days. Tired of strength-training with free weights? Check out a Pilates class, or hit the local climbing gym. There are so many ways to move your body that boredom should never push you back to the couch.

INSTEAD OF SKIPPING YOUR WORKOUT FOR WORK,

Turn your coffee breaks into fitness breaks. Stuck at your desk all day? I hear that. Here's what I do: Every few hours I get up from the computer and do 20 push-ups, 20 squats, and 20 backward-chair push-ups, and hold a 60-second plank. Then I quickly walk around the office for five minutes. If your work environment is a little more formal, get creative by taking a short walk outside every couple of hours, or spend five minutes out of every hour "sitting" without your chair.

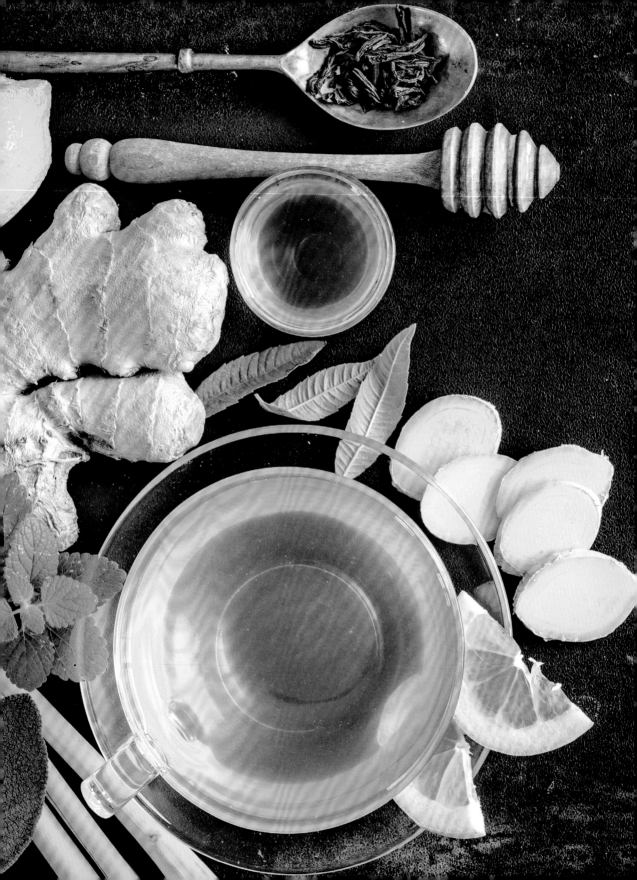

CHAPTER 3

Food to Fuel Your Life

"Let food be thy medicine and medicine be thy food."

—HIPPOCRATES

I love food. Always have. But I haven't always loved the kind of food that loves me back.

In my grade-school years, I started my day with Cap'n Crunch cereal, lunched on white-bread sandwiches slathered with sugary peanut butter and jam, and snacked on Entenmann's cakes—washed down with Coca-Cola. Most of my dinners were home-cooked and pretty healthy, but I much preferred the Friday nights when Grandma took a break from the kitchen and my mother let us eat Swanson's TV dinners right off the trays while we watched *The Addams Family.* Such bliss!

In retrospect, I realize my idea of a meal plan was pretty much a recipe for disaster, loaded with unhealthy processed foods, salt, sugar, and very few real nutrients. I can't say for sure what my health would be like right now if I was still eating that way. But I have a few clues thanks to modern research:

• Poor nutrition is a major factor in almost all of the most debilitating diseases that rob us of our quality of life—and often of life itself—including diabetes, heart disease, stroke, cancer, osteoporosis, and arthritis. It weakens our immune system, so we get sick more often and have a harder time recovering from illness and injury. But it also robs us of energy, contributes to depression and other mental illnesses, and can damage our vision. Adding insult to injury, a poor or unhealthy diet even damages our skin and hair.

• Research from the CDC has found that half of American adults have at least one diet-related chronic disease, including diabetes, heart disease, and obesity. That's scary!

• Other CDC studies have found that two out of three Americans over age 20 are overweight, including 34.7 percent who are clinically obese. That's double the percentage of Americans who were obese 50 years ago. And the numbers are even higher for people between 40 and 59, of whom 39.5 percent are obese. While healthy people come in all shapes and sizes, people who gain more weight than their bodies can handle are at much greater risk of serious diseases and debilitating conditions, like joint and back pain.

• A World Health Organization review of over a thousand studies, which was published in the *New England Journal of Medicine* in 2016, found that obesity is strongly linked to at least 13 kinds of cancer, including cancers of the breast, uterus, ovaries, and pancreas.

• A study published in the *New England Journal of Medicine* in 2003 found that obesity could account for 20 percent of all cancer deaths in women 50 and older. In men, obesity may account for 14 percent of cancer deaths.

• You're at an even higher risk for health problems if you carry that weight around your belly, which may mean visceral fat has snuck in between your internal organs. Visceral fat is a particularly pernicious accumulation and is strongly linked to type 2 diabetes and other diseases.

The Weight-Loss Industry Is Losing, Too

After years of making money from people who want to lose weight, diet products and services are now losing customers. Seems more of us are changing our focus from the quick fix and toward lifelong healthy-eating choices. Could it be we're finally ready to believe all the evidence showing that fad diets just don't work?

Well ... maybe. Plenty of us still join the club. In 2014 there were about 108 million dieters in the United States, 82 percent of whom tried to lose weight by jumping from fad diet to fad diet.

The good news: The use of diet pills, foods, and programs has decreased drastically since 2007. The number of women reporting that they are currently on a diet has dropped 13 percent over the past two decades, according to market research company NPD Group. Now, women report they are interested in healthy eating and overall fitness to lose and maintain weight. Great news!

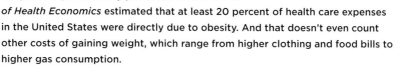

- Extra weight is bad for your brain, too. Research shows that people who are obese in midlife are at greater risk of developing Alzheimer's at a younger age.

- And all this weight isn't just unhealthy—it's also expensive. In 2008 the CDC estimated the medical costs of obesity in the United States were more than $147 billion. The same study found that average annual medical expenses for people who are obese were $1,429 higher than for people of normal weight. A separate study published in the *Journal of Health Economics* estimated that at least 20 percent of health care expenses in the United States were directly due to obesity. And that doesn't even count other costs of gaining weight, which range from higher clothing and food bills to higher gas consumption.

- The crazy thing is that despite all the extra eating we're doing, many of us still aren't getting the critical nutrients our bodies need to stay strong and healthy, which means that we get sick more often and age faster than we should. A 2015 report from the U.S. Department of Agriculture (USDA) found that many Americans are missing out on key vitamins including A, C, D, and E, as well as not getting enough folate, calcium, magnesium, potassium, iron, or fiber in their diets. We are, however, eating way too much salt and saturated fat, which are major culprits in heart disease and obesity.

- While exercise is important and helps to keep weight stable, large-scale studies have demonstrated that exercise alone isn't enough to reduce weight. What is? Eating fewer empty calories.

Here's the Plain Truth

What you eat can either shove you onto the fast track to old age—and possibly obesity—or lead you onto the path of a long, healthy life. And the difference is in the small choices you make every day.

Unfortunately, our society's relationship with food not only makes it easy to become simultaneously overweight, unhealthy, and undernourished but also makes it hard to develop better eating habits later in life.

Still, hard isn't the same as impossible. And there are lots of reasons—besides weight loss—for wanting to eat the kinds of food that love you back. Good food can give us more energy, better sleep, a smarter brain, clearer skin, stronger bones, and shinier

> ## "One cannot think well, love well, sleep well, if one has not dined well."
> —VIRGINIA WOOLF

hair. It can also slow down aging and protect us from more diseases than I can list. It is, truly, the right medicine for what's ailing so many of us.

Taking the Long View

By my unscientific estimate, 98.9 percent of books about food are—let's admit it—diet books. And while, yes, the majority of us could stand to shed some pounds, that isn't the goal of this chapter. However, it can be a perk. If you eat for health and longevity, weight loss is one likely side effect.

A healthy eating plan needs to be a long-term commitment, not a quick fix. So let's think about food as what it is: the source of all the delicious and nutritious energy we need to achieve our real goals of living well and living long.

Please note: Check with your physician before making any major changes to your diet, especially if you have existing health concerns. I encourage you to do your own research and get informed so you can decide what works best for your body, lifestyle, and goals.

What to Eat? That's Easy!

Here are the basic food habits we all need to cultivate:

Keep it real. The key to healthy eating is to start with foods that are as close as possible to the way they came out of the ground, off the tree, or from the sea or farm. These so-called whole foods have the most nutrients and the fewest additives. The fresher the food, the better the flavor, texture, and nutrition. The rule of thumb in the grocery store is to stick to the perimeter, where you'll find fresh produce, eggs, fish, and meat, and to be careful about the center, where most of the processed foods hang out. If you're buying packaged foods, get in the habit of reading every label to check ingredients and nutrition information—look for whole foods and be wary of any ingredients you can't pronounce.

Start (and end) with plants. Most nutritionists and longevity experts agree: More than half of our daily calories should come from plant-based sources (think veggies, legumes, grains, fruit, nuts, and seeds). To repeat: Plants should constitute *at least* 50 percent of your calories. We humans evolved to eat a wide variety of plants, and they provide us with an impressive array of vitamins and phytonutrients, plus complex carbohydrates, essential minerals, protein, and fiber. So add green to your plate!

Put protein in proportion. Protein is a primary component of our cells and a backup energy source. It's also critical to maintaining muscle mass as we age. In general, protein should make up 20 percent of the calories in our diet, regardless of source—but aim for proteins that don't come bundled with excess fat. If you eat meat, choose fish, poultry, and lean cuts of red meat. A mix of whole grains, nuts, and legumes will also provide complete protein. Natural nut butters—without added sugar—are great, too. Eggs are a good source of complete protein and important nutrients and, although the yolks are high in cholesterol, eggs are considered a healthy option for most people. If you have high cholesterol or heart disease, the American

What, Exactly, Is a Complete Protein?

Proteins are composed of amino acids. The human body needs a daily supply of nine different amino acids in certain proportions in order to function properly. A single food source that includes all nine in the appropriate ratio is considered a complete protein. Most animal-based protein (from meat, fish, poultry, egg, and dairy sources) is complete, while most plant-based protein is incomplete in one or more amino acids. Plant foods, however, can be combined in order to supplement each other with the missing amino acids. For instance, red beans with rice, pinto beans on corn tortillas, and peanut butter on whole wheat bread all provide complete proteins by pairing legumes with grains. *Tip:* Any diet that includes a variety of protein sources throughout the day, including whole grains and lean meats or fish, will provide adequate amino acids for most people.

Fat: A Primer

There are several kinds of fat found in foods, and each behaves differently in our bodies, so it's important to understand which is which.

• **Saturated fats** are made up of carbon atoms that are "saturated" with hydrogen atoms. They're often called "bad fats" because they raise our cholesterol, especially LDL cholesterol, and have been strongly linked with heart disease. In concentrated form, these fats are usually solid at room temperature, like butter or lard, but saturated fats are also found in animal products, like meat, cheese, cream, and eggs, as well as in coconuts and palm oil.

• **Unsaturated fats** have fewer hydrogen atoms than saturated fats and can be either monounsaturated (two fewer hydrogen atoms) or polyunsaturated (four fewer). Both types can lower overall cholesterol levels if you swap them for saturated fats, and monounsaturated fats may even increase "good" HDL cholesterol. As a rule, foods high in unsaturated fats are liquid at room temperature, like olive or canola oil, but foods like nuts, avocados, fish, and soybeans are also rich in unsaturated fats.

• **Trans fats, hydrogenated fats, and partially hydrogenated fats** may be the worst of the worst. They don't occur in nature but are made by adding hydrogen atoms to unsaturated oils in order to keep them solid at room temperature, as in margarine and other processed foods. They raise your bad cholesterol, lower your good cholesterol, and increase your risk of heart disease, which is why many trans fats have been banned from commercial food preparation. Steer clear.

• **Cholesterol** is a waxy substance our bodies use to build cells, make hormones, and even to make vitamin D. It has two basic forms—LDL and HDL—and we need both. But too much LDL can clog arteries, leading to high blood pressure, atherosclerosis (hardening of the arteries), heart disease, and stroke. Since our bodies make all the cholesterol we need, eating too much saturated or trans fat—which triggers the liver to up cholesterol production—raises levels of LDL. While eating cholesterol-laden foods also raises our levels, many recent studies have found that it has a much smaller effect than eating saturated or trans fats. *Tip:* All animal-based foods contain some cholesterol, but plant-based foods have none.

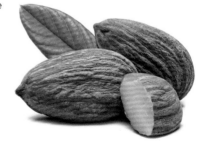

Heart Association recommends that you eat no more than two egg yolks per week, but you can enjoy as many egg whites as you wish.

Don't fear the fat. Our bodies and brains need fat to function and to absorb many of the other nutrients we need, so fat should make up about 30 percent of your calories in each meal. However, keep in mind that fat is high in caloric content, at nine calories per gram, so a little goes a long way. Most plant-based fats, like olive oil and avocados, are healthy, natural sources of unsaturated fat. However, the fats in dairy and most meats are usually the "bad" saturated kind, so use them sparingly for flavor rather than as the center of your meal.

Make friends with fiber. Fiber may be the secret weapon in the fight against diet-related diseases. It makes us feel full with fewer calories and keeps our digestive tract humming along. Fiber also lowers our cholesterol levels and stabilizes our blood sugar levels, thus reducing our risk of diabetes and heart disease. Eating a wide variety of fiber sources helps keep our intestinal bacteria healthy, and there's even evidence that fiber can reduce blood pressure and inflammation. Women age 50 and under should aim to consume 25 grams per day, while women 51 and over need about 21 grams daily. The best part? Fiber comes free with delicious veggies, fruits, and whole grains.

No more empty calories. Thanks to the rise in processed food, the U.S. Food and Drug Administration (FDA) has found most of us eat

How Much Is Too Much?

Portion sizes have gotten out of control in this country, where restaurants and food producers have promoted "bigger is better" slogans for years. The National Institute on Aging put together this handy cheat sheet to help us visualize and estimate healthy portion sizes.

One serving is about the same size as ...
- 1 cup of leafy greens, grains, or potato = a baseball
- 1 cup of fruit or ice cream = half a baseball
- 1 pancake or tortilla = a DVD
- 3 ounces of fish, meat, or poultry = a deck of cards
- 1½ ounces of cheese = four dice
- 2 tablespoons of nut butter = a Ping-Pong ball
- 1 teaspoon of butter = the tip of your index finger

more calories than we need while still not getting enough nutrients to be healthy. A woman over 50 of average height (five feet four inches) should consume about 1,800 calories per day—anyone who is significantly taller or more active may need more, while smaller women or anyone trying to lose weight will need fewer. So since we're trying to make sure we get maximum vitamins, minerals, and phytonutrients in our diets without gaining unnecessary weight, we want to choose foods that give us the most nutritional bang for our calorie bucks.

The First Step to Eating Well?

It's a simple recipe: Make plants the star of every meal, and turn everything else into supporting players. Plants provide the most of the good stuff: vitamins, minerals, complex carbohydrates, fiber, healthy protein, and unsaturated fats. They also have the least of the bad stuff: cholesterol and saturated fats. It's no coincidence that life expectancies are longer in countries like Greece, Italy, and Spain, which follow a "Mediterranean diet," based on fresh vegetables, fruits, legumes, nuts, and whole grains, with small amounts of dairy, fish, and meat. In the United States, the National Institutes of Health designed a similar eating plan to help people reduce their blood pressure. Turns out, the plan, Dietary Approaches to Stop Hypertension (DASH), has also reduced the risk of metabolic syndrome, heart disease, and other chronic diseases. But you don't need to follow a formal diet plan to improve your health; you just need to eat more plants. Here's your guide:

EAT THESE EVERY DAY:

Vegetables. Low in calories but high in phytonutrients, vitamins, minerals, fiber, and flavor, vegetables should occupy the majority of the plate in every meal. As a rule, more color equals more nutrients, so eat a wide variety of veggies daily. Artichokes, asparagus, beets, broccoli, cabbage, chard, kale, kelp, sweet potatoes, and spinach are especially nutrient-rich. Aim for at least two and a half to three and a half cups of vegetables every day.

Fruits. Since fruit can be high in calories, two or three servings per day is plenty, but it should still be an essential part of your diet because it is packed with

Follow Your Gut to Better Health

If you think your body is composed just of your own cells, think again. There are millions of tiny microorganisms living on and inside you, especially in your gastrointestinal tract. These "friendly bacteria" play critical roles in absorbing nutrients and allowing you to maintain a healthy weight. What's more, about 70 percent of our immune system actually lives in our gut tissue, so we want to keep our intestines healthy—including the resident bacteria! However, because we usually think of bacteria as bad, most of us don't take care of our helpful internal microbes as well as we should.

The result?

More than 70 million Americans have some kind of gut issue, such as irritable bowel syndrome, food allergies, bloating, gas, or constipation. Some of the suffering is caused when we develop sensitivity to foods like gluten or dairy, but research also shows that antibiotics are a major source of gut problems. Ingesting antibiotics, even in low doses, kills some of these good bacteria along with the bad and upsets the overall balance of the gut microbiome, disrupting our digestion and our internal weight-regulation system. Just one course of antibiotics can create long-term changes in the balance of good and bad bacteria, so to protect your internal microbiome, follow these simple steps:

• Say no to antibiotics if you have a cold or any other viral infection. Viruses aren't bacteria, so antibiotics are of no use against them.

• Choose only antibiotic-free meat to avoid ingesting residual antibiotics.

• Eat fermented and cultured foods, like sauerkraut, kimchi, miso, kefir, and unsweetened yogurt. They contain friendly bacteria—also called probiotics—that may help restore your internal balance.

• Pop a probiotic pill every day—but check with your PCP first about which type and dosage are appropriate for you, especially if you have a compromised immune system.

• Eat lots of fiber, which is a great food source for the helpful microbes inside us. When we feed them well, they stay healthy and, in turn, so do we. The best sources of fiber are vegetables, legumes, and fruits.

• Stay hydrated. Like you, microbes need water, too!

Healthy Snacks to Make, Not Buy

These treats are lower than their store-bought counterparts in sodium, sugar, fat, calories, and cost! Plus, they're supereasy to make.

IF YOU LOVE GRANOLA BARS,
Mix 2 cups of uncooked oats with ¾ cup of honey, plus a handful of nuts and raisins, a sprinkle of cinnamon, and (optional) up to ½ cup of unsweetened coconut. Spread the mixture on a sheet pan and refrigerate it for an hour or two until solid, then cut it into bars. Store the bars chilled.

IF YOU LOVE FROZEN YOGURT,
Stir a bit of honey and 2 teaspoons of unsweetened cocoa powder into Greek yogurt.

IF YOU LOVE NACHOS,
That makes two of us! Sprinkle 4 ounces of multigrain chips with 2 to 3 ounces of grated cheese and bake at 425°F for six minutes.

IF YOU LOVE FRENCH FRIES,
Slice up a sweet potato and toss the wedges with a little olive oil, then sprinkle with salt and pepper. Bake at 450°F for 20 minutes, tossing halfway through.

IF YOU LOVE BLENDED COFFEE DRINKS,
Skip the barista. Blend 2 cups of strong cold coffee with ¼ cup milk or unsweetened nut milk, 1 to 2 teaspoons of honey to taste, a dash of vanilla extract, and ice. Add 2 tablespoons of cocoa powder to make it a mocha!

IF YOU LOVE MOVIE POPCORN,
Put 1½ tablespoons of popcorn kernels in a microwave-safe bowl, cover the bowl with a plate, and microwave for two to four minutes—no oil needed! Sprinkle with a little grated Parmesan. Alternatively, try an air popper.

IF YOU LOVE POTATO CHIPS,
Sprinkle kale leaves with olive oil and salt, and bake them on a tray at 250°F for 10 to 15 minutes. Same crunch, fewer calories.

vitamins, minerals, and lots of fiber. Raspberries, blueberries, cranberries, oranges, grapefruit, cantaloupe, tomatoes (yes, a tomato is a fruit!), and—believe it or not—watermelon are among the nutritional standouts in the fruit department, but seek a variety for balance.

Legumes. Beans and legumes, like lentils, split peas, kidney beans, and especially black beans, are great sources of protein, complex carbohydrates, fiber, and essential nutrients. Eat a half cup to one cup of cooked beans or legumes per day, preferably in combination with a healthy carb, like brown rice or whole wheat bread, to form a complete protein. Add a serving of veggies and you've got yourself a nutritious and delicious meal.

Nuts and seeds. They're high in protein, fiber, minerals, and heart-healthy fats. Eat two servings a day, preferably raw or dry-roasted rather than salted or sugared. Standouts include walnuts, peanuts, pistachios, almonds, and sunflower seeds—but you really can't go wrong as long as you keep portions in control and skip the salt. One serving is about a quarter cup of nuts or two tablespoons of nut butter (choose natural nut butters with no added sugar). *Bonus:* They're delicious, nutritious, and portable—perfect for a midafternoon snack on the go or at the office.

What's the Deal With Dairy?

As we get older, our ability to digest dairy—commonly called lactose tolerance—may be diminished, and some of us experience intestinal woes as a result.

We absolutely need calcium to keep our bones dense as we get older and should eat calcium-rich foods daily. But contrary to popular belief, not all of the best sources of calcium are dairy. Yogurt is great, but so are other sources such as sardines, almonds, dark leafy greens, broccoli, blackstrap molasses, tofu, salmon, and calcium-enriched nut milks.

Dairy products, therefore, are not specifically recommended, except yogurt, which contains beneficial bacteria that break down lactose for us. If you do eat dairy, remember that most cheeses are high in saturated fat and should be used as a topping, not a meal. Likewise, a splash of half-and-half in your coffee is fine, but a bowl of cream-based soup should be a very occasional indulgence.

Olive oil. Extra-virgin olive oil is an especially healthy fat, because it contains loads of phytonutrients and can lower cholesterol. Use it in place of butter in cooking, and drizzle it on salads and vegetables instead of cream-based sauces. For baking, try light olive oil, which imparts very little flavor, or swap in another unsaturated oil, like canola. Other good options include

Food Habits for an Ageless Glow From Head to Toe

Beauty really does start on the inside. And you can boost it by making sure these nutrient-rich ingredients find a place on your plate several times a week.

For Your Hair

• Spinach and kale are rich in vitamins that give you a healthy scalp and strong roots.
• Sweet potatoes and other orange fruits and vegetables contain vitamin A, which makes hair shine.
• Peanuts, pine nuts, sunflower seeds, hazelnuts, and other nuts and seeds will give your scalp a vitamin E boost to improve circulation and hair growth.

For Your Skin and Lips

• Avocados are rich in hydrating monounsaturated fat.
• Our bodies use the vitamin C in citrus, tomatoes, and bell peppers to make collagen, the protein that keeps our skin supple.
• Walnuts offer omega-3s to help replenish skin cells.

• Grapes are rich in resveratrol, which may counter the effects of UV radiation. But make sure to enjoy this fruit mostly in its unfermented form, as too much alcohol dehydrates your skin and makes it harder for your liver to filter out toxins, which could in turn trigger skin problems.

For Your Nails

• Eggs supply lots of biotin, which strengthens hair and nails.
• The magnesium in almonds and the zinc in oysters are important for helping your body make proteins, including those that build strong nails.

For Your Metabolism

• Dark chocolate helps burn fat and slows the intake of sugar into your blood cells.
• Oats boost metabolism and protect you from blood sugar spikes, as do bananas—especially if they're a little green.
• Grapefruit lowers insulin and helps to regulate fat storage.

> # *Eat food. Not too much. Mostly plants."*
> —MICHAEL POLLAN

walnut, sesame, avocado, and peanut oils. Aim to consume about five to six teaspoons per day of any healthy oil.

Whole grains. Grains like whole wheat, brown rice, oats, barley, and quinoa are rich sources of complex carbohydrates and fiber, as well as certain proteins that are missing from legumes. Eat two to three servings a day. One serving is a slice of whole wheat or multigrain bread, a cup of cooked oatmeal or pasta, or a half cup of cooked brown rice.

EAT THESE THREE TIMES A WEEK:

Fish. Aim to eat a three- to four-ounce serving of fish three times per week. But be smart: Choose fish that aren't exposed to high levels of mercury. Salmon is well-known as a superfood, but small fish like anchovies and sardines are also good choices, as are mackerel and cod. *Bonus:* Fatty fish, like arctic char and lake trout, contain loads of omega-3 acids, which have proven health benefits, especially for your heart.

Eggs. Eggs are high in protein, vitamins, minerals, and omega-3s. As mentioned earlier, they are also high in cholesterol, but for most of us the nutritional benefits outweigh any negatives. Serve eggs alongside whole grains and vegetables for a balanced meal full of protein, carbs, and fats.

Yogurt. Natural and Greek yogurt (plain yogurt that's been strained to make it thicker) are fantastic foods. They're loaded with calcium, protein, and helpful bacteria and are usually fine even for people who are lactose-intolerant. Yogurt makes a terrific breakfast, lunch, or snack option with fruit or granola. It can also be used in place of sour cream, butter, or cheese in toppings and sauces. To avoid hidden calories, choose only unsweetened varieties with no additives. If you like flavored yogurt, start with plain and drizzle on a little honey or maple syrup, or mix with natural fruit preserves.

Avocados. Technically a fruit, the avocado deserve a category of its own. It's high in calories but also rich in healthy fats and complex carbs, so enjoy an avocado two or three times a week. One of my favorite quick breakfasts is to mash up some avocado with plain Greek yogurt, a little sea salt, a drop of olive oil, and a sprinkle of cumin, and spread it on whole grain toast—with or without an egg on top for a protein boost.

Poultry. While plant-based proteins are lower in fat and calories, eating poultry two or three times a week is fine. As with fish, a serving size is three to four ounces, uncooked. And remember that skinless cuts are much lower in fat.

Dark chocolate. If you have a hankering for something sweet, dip into your stash of dark chocolate (at least 70 percent cacao). Unlike most candies, or milk and white chocolate, dark chocolate packs a nice dose of nutrients

Grocery Cheat Sheet: Always Keep These On Hand

If you stock your pantry with these basics, you'll have a head start in making simple, nutritious meals:

• Brown rice—there are many varieties to explore!
• Whole grain pastas
• Oatmeal
• Quinoa
• Plain canned and dried beans—try black beans, kidney beans, and garbanzo beans for starters
• Dried lentils and split peas
• Red wine vinegar
• Apple cider vinegar

• Balsamic vinegar
• Olive oil
• Sea salt
• Canned tomatoes
• Dried herbs, like basil, thyme, and dill
• Spices like cinnamon, chili powder, red pepper flakes, and freshly ground black pepper
• Honey
• Maple syrup
• Fresh parsley
• Lemons and limes
• Unsweetened plain or Greek yogurt
• Canned salmon and sardines

Set Yourself Up for Success

For a lot of us, it can seem easier to eat junk food than healthy food. To create better long-term habits, look for ways to turn that equation around.

Invest in storage containers. Plastic or glass containers with secure lids are invaluable for healthy eating. Use them to portion dinner leftovers for lunch, stash precooked grains and beans for another meal, and bring yogurt, hummus, nuts, or other snacks with you to work. A small cooler makes a great tote to keep things cool until lunchtime.

Buy some good knives and keep them sharp. If there's one downside to cooking with veggies, it's that there can be a lot of chopping. But good tools go a long way in making food prep fast and easy. You don't need a whole set of cutlery, just a sturdy chef's knife, a paring knife, and a veggie peeler. Pair them

with some sturdy plastic cutting boards and you're set. Wood cutting boards, while beautiful, can trap germs and bacteria because they're harder to wash. *Tip:* Dedicate one cutting board to stinky stuff, like garlic and onions—and make sure you have a board big enough to whack open a whole squash, too.

Buy—and use—a couple of good veggie-focused cookbooks. Even dedicated carnivores can get great recipes from vegetarian cookbooks. The authors are full of advice on how to build delicious, balanced meals from plants (and it won't hurt their feelings if you throw some fish on the side). For starters, check out Deborah Madison's *The New Vegetarian Cooking for Everyone,* Mark Bittman's *How to Cook Everything Vegetarian*, and just about anything from Mollie Katzen, including *Vegetable Heaven.*

and antioxidants. But don't go crazy—a healthy serving size is 1.5 ounces. With most bars, that works out to roughly a one-and-a-half-inch square.

EAT THESE ONCE A WEEK OR LESS:

Cake, cookies, pie, and ice cream. Dessert. Sure, enjoy it once in a while. But not every day and not as a mindless snack. Opt for homemade and steer clear of the packaged stuff. Also keep portion size in mind. Most of us have gotten so used to these oversized, oversweetened "goodies" that our taste buds are out of whack. But we can reset our palates so we don't crave so much sugar and instead enjoy it as an occasional extravagance.

Food for Thought

There's no doubt that if you want to live a long and healthy life, one of the best things you can do is eat a balanced diet full of plants and whole foods. But many scientists who study the effect of nutrition on long-term health have started to suggest that every now and then, you need to eat almost nothing at all.

One of the best known fasting researchers is Valter Longo, who is the director of the University of Southern California Longevity Institute and a pioneer in researching the impact of food on life expectancy. Longo and other researchers, including Mark Mattson, a neuroscientist at the National Institute on Aging, have conducted a number of studies on rodents and humans that suggest that occasional controlled semi-fasting can slow down aging, shed fat, improve heart health, build the immune system, ward off dementia, speed up generation of new cells, reduce inflammation, recalibrate insulin, lower cholesterol and blood pressure, and possibly fight certain cancers.

Wow! Who knew so little (food, that is) could do so much?

As Longo explains it, our body accumulates "junk" over time, which can prematurely age us and make us feel worn down and tired. By occasionally restricting our food intake, he says we can effectively shed the junk and restore ourselves to better health.

However, researchers like Longo caution against a complete fast, which can be very dangerous outside of a doctor's supervision, and also against long-term caloric restriction, which is not considered safe or effective in promoting health.

On the other hand, periodic bouts of semi-fasting, where you eat small amounts of food and drink plenty of water and herbal teas for a specific period of time, may offer promising potential. There is increasing evidence that during a short-term semi-fast some pretty amazing things happen:

OLD CELLS GET BOOTED OFF THE ISLAND. Autophagy (from a Greek term meaning "self-eating") is a process by which our bodies clear out aged and diseased cells, many of which could mutate into cancer or immunological diseases, and may even play a role in aging. In 2016 the Nobel Prize in Physiology or Medicine was awarded to Yoshinori Ohsumi, the Japanese biologist whose work in understanding autophagy may provide a path to preventing or even curing certain illnesses. And restricting calories for a short time seems to be the most effective method of triggering autophagy.

YOUR IMMUNE SYSTEM GETS A BOOST. White blood cells are produced at a higher rate after a short fast, strengthening the entire immune system.

YOU LOWER IGF-1 LEVELS. IGF-1 is a growth hormone. It's essential when we're young, but as we get older, high levels of IGF-1 may make us more susceptible to cancer and accelerate aging. Fasting lowers IGF-1 levels very quickly. However, levels will eventually go back up when you resume normal eating, so for a sustained benefit, you need to commit to fasting periodically.

CHEMOTHERAPY MAY WORK BETTER. Some research has shown that occasional semi-fasting may be able to "starve" cancer cells while simultaneously protecting healthy cells from chemotherapy toxicity.

CANCER RISK MAY BE REDUCED. An intriguing study published in *JAMA Oncology* reported that breast cancer survivors between the ages of 27 and 70 who simply "fasted" for 13 hours or more during the night (between dinner and breakfast) reduced the risk of having their early-stage breast cancer come back. Those who went longer than 13 hours between meals showed even lower measurements of the biomarkers associated with cancer risk.

There are still many questions about how fasting works, including establishing the optimal time between meals to trigger the "fasting" response. While a 2014 study from the National Academy of Sciences acknowledges that the contemporary three square meals a day is abnormal from an evolutionary perspective, research conducted with both animal and human participants showed that food-restriction periods of as little as 16 hours (which can be accomplished by combining an early dinner and a late breakfast) can improve health.

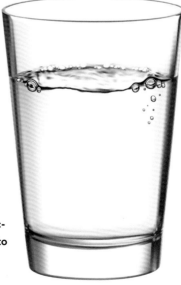

Of course, a fast will help only if you eat well regularly. If you're considering a semi-fast, the most important rule is: Talk with your doctor! Medical supervision is essential, especially if you fast for over 24 hours. Never consider a water-only fast. And fasting is never okay for someone who is pregnant or lactating; is a type 1 diabetic; is under 18; has or has ever had an eating disorder; or has a BMI of 18.5 or lower.

Don't confuse intermittent fasting with daily caloric restriction. This approach is intended to be an occasional event to help boost your health only if it is appropriate for you. It should not be a daily occurrence.

A Lot From a Little:
My Experiment With Fasting

There are several approaches to semi-fasting, including the 5:2 plan and alternate-day fasting, popularized by Michael Mosley and Krista Varady, respectively. For my own experiment, I decided to try Longo's five-day fast, which relies on carefully portioned and nutritionally balanced foods designed to trick the body into thinking it's truly fasting. In fact, I was eating throughout the day, albeit in small amounts. Surprisingly, I wasn't hungry at all and had more than enough energy to exercise, work, and carry on with my day. I even slept more soundly.

Because I had never tried it before, Longo suggested that I repeat the five-day fast once a month for three months and then fast just two or three times a year as maintenance. After three months and three rounds of the program, I had lost an extra eight pounds I'd been dragging around, including an inch around my waist, where the evil visceral fat is stored.

But here's the real payoff: I had blood tests done before I started my first fast and then again after the third fast. The prefasting blood work showed an elevation in certain inflammation markers—definitely a cause for concern—but the postfasting tests showed a significant decrease in these same markers.

White stuff. Reduce the amount of empty calories you eat and keep your blood sugar levels balanced by swapping the "white stuff"—white rice, white bread, white pasta, white sugar, white potatoes—for whole wheat, whole grains, brown rice, sweet potatoes, and healthy sweeteners. It's not necessary to eliminate white stuff completely, but when it comes to food, more color usually means more nutrients. And more nutrients mean better health.

Fruit juice. We're talking a small (three-quarter-cup) serving of 100 percent fruit juice—not sweetened "fruit drink." Fruit juice is mostly fruit sugar without the fiber or complex carbs you'd get from eating whole fruit. However, juice does offer some vitamins and can make a tasty pick-me-up now and then. For the most benefits, choose fresh-squeezed and leave the pulp in.

Red meat. Sorry, Dr. Atkins, but most research says the best plan for long-term health is to limit your intake of animal protein overall—specifically from red meat (beef, lamb, and pork). Why? Even lean cuts are high in saturated fat and cholesterol compared with other protein sources. But if you intend to keep meat in your life, eat it only on occasion, in three- to four-ounce servings, and choose antibiotic-free sources.

WASH IT DOWN WITH:

Water. Make it your drink of choice. Some research has promoted the idea that eight glasses a day is ideal, while other studies suggest there's no magic number. The bottom line? Drink what you need to stay hydrated. Regular water intake is necessary for basic body functions, and dehydration is a common cause of headaches and constipation. How do you know if you're dehydrated? Check the color of your urine. If it's dark, start chugging. By the way, there's no special benefit to bottled water, so tap is fine. Add a slice of lemon or lime for flavor.

Herbal tea. Hot or chilled, caffeine-free herbal teas are a great way to stay hydrated and keep your stomach feeling full. Mint, chamomile, ginger, licorice, and hibiscus are great starters, but there are plenty of other options, depending on your taste.

Green tea. A cup or two of hot or cold green tea per day will give you hefty doses of antioxidants. Keep a container of green tea with mint leaves in the fridge for a refreshing alternative to sweetened beverages or sodas. But remember: Green tea still has caffeine!

Coffee and black tea. Starting your morning with two to three cups of coffee or black tea (not a sugary mochaccino) has been shown to offer real health benefits, both physically and mentally. But don't

To Keep Weight in Check, Weigh In Every Day

Tracking your pounds can be a simple but effective way to monitor your body. Tech lovers can find scales that sync wirelessly with phone health apps, but an old-school notebook works just as well. If, however, you have an eating disorder or find that the daily weigh-in is causing you stress, ditch the scale and focus on other measurements, like energy level and how your body feels.

keep pouring—too much caffeine can lead to health problems ranging from dehydration to high blood pressure to osteoporosis. And, of course, it can keep you up at night.

Red wine. Red wine offers significant quantities of the antiaging power-house resveratrol, and a five-ounce glass with a meal several times a week has been shown to have many health benefits. Sadly, research on potential benefits of white wine and beer has been inconclusive. If you drink alcohol,

How to Be an Angel While Eating Out

A recent study conducted at Duke University found that merely listing a salad on a restaurant menu could cause people to add French fries to their order. Just knowing that we have the option of a good choice apparently makes our brain feel justified in making a bad one. Go figure!

A similar brain trick, known as the health halo, leads us to eat larger portions and more fattening sides and desserts if restaurants label our entrée as "healthy." Be smarter than your brain! Start with a salad or vegetable as an appetizer. Opt for sautéed, grilled, or roasted items, rather than fried. Order sauces and dressings on the side, so you can add just a bit.

And resist the impulse to clean your plate! If anything is bigger than a proper serving size, cut it down and push the extra to the side right away. In general, plan on eating half of what you're served, and either share the rest with a companion or take it home for another meal.

When it comes time for dessert, skip the sweets and order an after-dinner tea. Sipping a hot cup of an herbal brew, like mint or ginger, can help with digestion.

If you crave something sweet on the side, try a square of nutrition-packed dark chocolate. If you must splurge, get a small serving and savor every bite. This is the not-so-secret secret behind the dining traditions in countries like France, Spain, Italy, Germany, Norway, Sweden, and Finland—all of which have longer life expectancies than the United States.

And if you still have trouble with portion control, ask for a salad plate. Eating off a smaller plate can help you keep your portion sizes in perspective.

red wine is clearly the healthiest choice, but excess consumption is always going to do more harm than good, so stick to one glass.

JUST SAY NO TO:

Processed foods. If you start reading the labels at the grocery store, you'll soon see a string of ingredients that sure didn't come from Grandma's cookbook. These unpronounceable things are called additives, because they aren't actually food but compounds and chemicals added to make food last longer on the shelf or to change its flavor, color, or texture. They include preservatives, like potassium sorbate and sodium benzoate; sweeteners, like high-fructose corn syrup and glucose; and flavor enhancers, like monosodium glutamate and hydrolyzed soy protein. Not all additives are bad for you (although some surely are), but none of them are *good* for you, either. And if you're chowing down on poly-sorba-gluta-whatever, then you aren't eating the things that would actually feed your cells and help your body take care of itself. You are, however, getting a lot of empty calories and excess sodium along the way. So as hard as it might be in the beginning, we have got to ditch the factory-made foods. This includes processed meats, frozen TV dinners, cookies, chips, snacks—all of it.

Sugary drinks. Soda, syrupy coffee concoctions, and other sweetened drinks are not your friends—especially when they're sweetened with high-fructose corn syrup. They're basically a low-quality dessert, but many of us drink them like, well ... water. We're chugging hundreds (or thousands) of empty calories every day, along with lots of artificial additives. These sugary drinks spike your blood sugar and may be a culprit in metabolic problems and diabetes, as well as obesity. And diet drinks are no improvement.

Artificially sweetened food and drinks. If there's anything worse than sugary sodas, it's sugar-free sodas. Same goes for "diet" foods. These foods don't help you lose weight. In fact, studies show they may hinder it. There is some evidence that artificial sweeteners may increase your cravings for junk food, stimulate fat storage, and have the same impact on insulin levels as sugar would.

Oh, and meanwhile they supply your body with regular doses of artificial chemicals. Yuck!

The Takeaway

After reading reams of research, changing my own food habits, and even experimenting with fasting, I have a much better understanding of the impact that food has on my body, energy level, weight, and overall long-term health and well-being. The evidence is clear: The better your diet, the better your life.

What's more, if you eat to *gain* health, then you're making a positive, life-affirming choice, which is pretty much the opposite of "dieting" to try to *lose* weight. As soon as you start obsessing over things that you "can't" or "shouldn't" eat, you set yourself up for misery. Food should nourish you, not punish you! After all, an occasional tasty cookie is just a tasty cookie, not cause for a guilt trip.

Achieving—and holding steady at—your body's healthiest weight is one nice benefit of eating well. But the greatest reward is a longer, fuller, more vibrant (and delicious) life.

15 Small Steps to Eating Healthy

❶ Eat a protein-packed breakfast.

❷ Eat at least three servings of veggies and two of fruit per day.

❸ Eat one serving of beans per day.

❹ Choose whole grains.

❺ Eat fish three times a week.

❻ Eat dairy and meat in small portions—or not at all.

❼ Cut back on sugar. Then go ahead and cut back some more.

❽ Enjoy dark chocolate up to three times a week.

❾ Cook dinner at home at least four times a week.

❿ Go for quality over quantity.

⓫ Choose minimally processed foods.

⓬ Read labels on packaged foods and avoid additives, added sugars, and words you don't recognize.

⓭ If you drink coffee, skip the sweeteners.

⓮ If you drink alcohol, stick to one glass of red wine per day.

⓯ Drink water all day, every day.

A Well-Fueled Life

Ready to make healthy eating a part of your long-term lifestyle?

INSTEAD OF TRYING TO CHANGE YOUR WHOLE DIET,

Ease into it. Small changes really do add up, so take it a little at a time. Start by getting portion sizes under control and by adding more veggies to every meal. If you still need to rely on prepared foods, choose those with fewer additives and less fat, salt, and sugar. Even if dinner is a microwave pizza, steam some veggies or make a salad to go with it. Heck, no matter what's for dinner (or lunch), make a salad to go with it.

INSTEAD OF TRYING TO FIGURE IT OUT ON THE FLY,

Make a meal plan. Carve out a half hour and plan your meals for the week—including snacks. Gather recipes, check the pantry, and make a grocery list. This little chore will pay you back a hundredfold by saving you money, smoothing out your weeknights, preventing food from going to waste, and keeping you on track.

INSTEAD OF EATING OUT,

Cook more. If you prepare more meals at home, you'll spend less money, eat more veggies, and control your intake of salt, sugar, and fats. If you don't cook much now, search out beginner-friendly websites and cookbooks and teach yourself a few simple dishes you can put into rotation. And remember: It doesn't have to be all-or-nothing. Pick up a rotisserie chicken to go with your home-cooked veggie dishes. That's fine!

INSTEAD OF SCRAMBLING AT DINNERTIME,

Make it ahead. Lean on foods you can cook in advance. Throw a stew into the Crock-Pot in the morning and, when you get home, just toss a salad, grab some tortillas, and you're done. Anytime you'll be home for a couple of hours, throw some dried beans on the stove to cook, then freeze them in two-cup portions to reheat later. Whenever you're cooking grains, stews, or soups, make double (or triple) batches and stash extra portions in the fridge or freezer to heat later on. The easier it is to access healthy food, the better you'll eat.

INSTEAD OF SKIMPING ON FRESH FOODS,

Go frozen. If your grocery store (or budget) doesn't provide a good variety of fresh vegetables and fruits, hit the freezer section for plain frozen broccoli, blueberries, and much more. Unlike canning, freezing preserves most of the flavor and nutrition of foods, without added salt or preservatives. Frozen fruits make for great smoothies. Freezing may change the texture of some vegetables, but they're still perfect for soups, stews, and purees. Just be sure to pick the fresh-frozen options, not those breaded, coated in cheese, or with other added ingredients.

INSTEAD OF MIDDAY MUNCHIES,

Treat snacks as real food. If you can easily skip the midday snacks, great. But if your blood sugar dips between meals, then include healthy snacks in your meal plan so afternoon hunger pangs don't drive you to the nearest vending machine. Try hummus and whole wheat pita wedges, celery sticks with peanut butter, or cucumbers with dill-yogurt dip (stir fresh or dried dill and a pinch of salt into a little Greek yogurt). If you're on the go, pack veggie sticks or fruit and nuts in your bag.

INSTEAD OF MINDLESS NIBBLING,

Keep a food journal. Studies show you'll eat better and consume fewer calories if you keep a journal of what you eat and drink. My wearable fitness band lets me track my meals and calculate my caloric and nutritional intake, but a simple notebook can be just as effective.

INSTEAD OF FOLLOWING THE FADS,

Listen to your body. Ever wonder why your girlfriend raves about the Paleo diet, but when you try it, you feel awful? Research shows that we all absorb and metabolize nutrients differently, based on our genetics, gut bacteria, body type—and even our exposure to chemicals. Pay attention to what makes you feel your best, and respect your body's specific needs.

INSTEAD OF GIVING IN TO CRAVINGS,

Check your mood. There's a lot of evidence that when people are stressed or unhappy, they'll try to boost their serotonin levels by chowing down on carbohydrates. This may improve your mood temporarily, but it's a recipe for overeating and won't solve your problems. If you're suddenly dreaming of a mac-and-cheese binge, calm down and evaluate your mood, and then eat a balanced meal. (But if you must indulge, at least choose a small portion and toss some greens on the side.) And if you're depressed for more than a couple of weeks, see a doctor.

INSTEAD OF BIG DINNERS,

Load up early. Try to get most of your calories early in the day. There's a wise old saying: "Eat like a king in the morning, a prince at midday, and a pauper at night." Not only do you need more energy during the day than you do when you're snoozing, but eating a hearty meal in the morning tends to reduce snacking and food cravings later in the day.

INSTEAD OF CARBO-LOADING AT BREAKFAST,

Start your day with protein. Recent studies have demonstrated that eating a sizable portion (25 to 35 grams) of protein in the morning makes us feel fuller and decreases snacking for the rest of the day. One 2008 study found that people on a weight-loss diet lost 65 percent more weight and decreased their waist size by an extra 34 percent if they started their day with two eggs five days a week instead of eating the same calories' worth of bagels.

INSTEAD OF COFFEE CONCOCTIONS,

Just drink coffee. There are plenty of benefits to a cuppa java, but most of the drinks at your local café are loaded with so much sugar they're best treated as dessert. Save yourself the calories and switch to an unsweetened brew—with a splash of milk or nut milk if you like. You can ease the transition by spooning a teaspoon of sugar into your mug, but cut the sweeteners out completely if you can.

INSTEAD OF CHUGGING SODA,

Choose sparkling water, a spritzer, or iced tea. If you love the bubbles in soda, choose unsweetened sparkling water or club soda instead. Add a slice of lemon or lime, or mix in a splash of fruit juice for a refreshing fruit spritzer. If it's the caffeine boost you're after, pour a glass of unsweetened iced green or black tea. But ditch the empty calories and chemicals, please.

INSTEAD OF DEFAULTING TO SUGAR,

Welcome the wide world of natural sweeteners. Maple syrup, honey, molasses, and agave nectar are all more nutritious and less stressful for your insulin levels than white sugar and its evil cousin, high-fructose corn syrup. Most recipes can be adapted to replace sugar, but aim to use fewer sweeteners overall.

INSTEAD OF SUPERSIZING IT,

Order smart when you dine out. Choose restaurants with an abundance of plant-based offerings (Mediterranean, Persian, Indian, Ethiopian, Thai, Vietnamese, and Japanese cuisines are good places to start), and remember that food eaten out is still going to end up in your body.

INSTEAD OF CHOWING SOLO,

Eat with other people. If you live with other people, then eat together daily. If not, invite friends over on a regular basis. Not only are shared meals important for emotional connection, but it's more efficient to plan, shop, and cook for a group than to dine alone. What's more, eating with others encourages us to make healthier choices—and we'll set a good example for our kids.

INSTEAD OF "LOW-FAT,"

Choose healthy fats in small amounts. Yes, excess saturated fats can be unhealthy, but overreaction to this risk has left many of us obsessed with processed "low-fat" foods. And that's created new problems as we end up eating too many sugars, starches, and additives instead. Skip the fake health foods and instead use modest portions of beneficial fats, like olive oil, to add flavor to your meals. If you're a bacon or cheese lover, buy the real thing, but sprinkle it on lightly.

INSTEAD OF COW'S MILK,

Try nut milks. Whether you're ditching dairy or just cutting back on saturated fat, almond, cashew, and soy milks can usually be used as a one-for-one replacement for milk. They're great in coffee and work well for baking, too. But read those labels! Choose unsweetened, calcium-enriched versions only. And while coconut milk is popular and does contain some useful nutrients, it has no protein and is very high in saturated fat and calories, so it's not the best option as a full-time milk substitute.

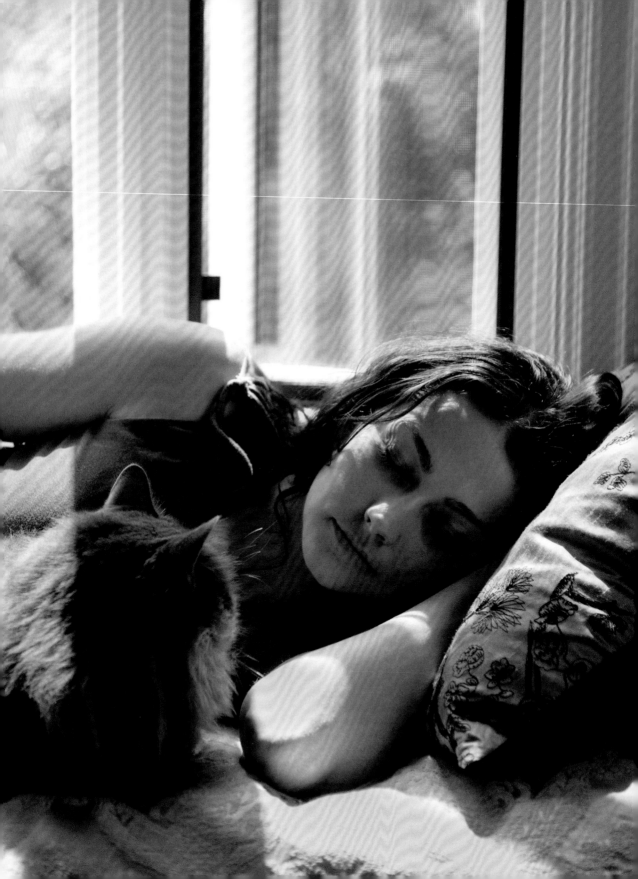

CHAPTER 4

Sleep, the Third Pillar of Health

"A good laugh and a long sleep are the best cures in the doctor's book."

—IRISH PROVERB

Oh, for the nights of long ago: rolling into bed after 2 a.m., then lingering in blissful sleep until noon. When my eyes fluttered open, I'd yawn, stretch, and maybe turn over for a little more shut-eye (or some sex before the shut-eye).

Now? Sleep is hard work. Most nights, I try everything in my power not to wake up at 3 a.m. and when that fails, I just hope to slip back into unconsciousness for a little longer. But I know it won't last. Even on the weekends, my eyelids pop open at 5:30 a.m., no matter how dark it is or how tired I am. And I can't blame these early wake-ups on the kids or dog (not all of them, anyway).

Arianna Huffington, media powerhouse and founder of *The Huffington Post,* has become a self-appointed spokeswoman for snoozing since the day several years

The High Price of Missing Sleep

Sleep disorders, sleep deprivation, and plain old sleepiness contribute over $15.9 billion to the national health care bill, and Americans spend nearly $41 billion annually on sleep aids and remedies. Add that to the estimated $411 billion a year in lost worker productivity in the United States and the $31 billion a year in insomnia-related accidents and it's clear we're spending a lot of $$$ on our lack of Z's.

> ## "*Renew your estranged relationship with sleep—you will be more productive, more effective, more creative, and more likely to enjoy your life.*"
> —ARIANNA HUFFINGTON

ago when she passed out from exhaustion and broke her cheekbone. She now claims to sleep at least eight hours every night *and* to nap during the day. She installed sleep pods in the office for employees and has written several editorials and books arguing for the importance of sleep for a well-lived life. She's my sleep idol.

It seems crazy that something as fundamental as sleep needs celebrity advocates, but in our current achievement-obsessed culture, many people brag about how little sleep they get—as if chronic exhaustion were a mark of success. We complain about the time we spend sleeping and imagine all the more exciting things we could do instead. And it's true. Compared to our go-go days, sleep can seem a tad underwhelming.

While it might not be exciting (well, depending on your dreams), we need sleep just as much as air, water, and food. In fact, it's the third pillar of health, along with good nutrition and regular exercise.

What's Going On Before the Alarm Goes Off?

Truth is, sleep time isn't wasted at all. Adequate rest is critical for optimal functioning of the immune system, brain health, hormone regulation, weight management, blood pressure, emotional well-being, and more.

Here are just a few of the things your body is doing while you're snoozing:

- **Cleaning your brain.** Like the rest of our bodies, our brains collect toxins during the day. As we sleep, our brain cells shrink temporarily, allowing cerebrospinal fluid to wash the toxins out into the circulatory system, which will carry them away. But if you don't sleep long enough or deeply enough, the process won't be as effective, potentially resulting in a buildup of detritus, including amyloid beta protein, which has been linked to Alzheimer's and dementia.

• **Keeping the pounds off.** No, not by tossing and turning. Sleep helps your body regulate many hormones, including those that control blood sugar and appetite. Research has repeatedly correlated inadequate sleep with metabolic problems, and in one small study healthy people were turned into near diabetics in less than one week simply by restricting their sleep to four and a half hours per night! Besides, you probably won't stick to your fitness routine if you're always exhausted.

• **Fighting infection.** Ever wonder why you want to curl up in bed at the first sign of an illness? Sleep boosts the immune system and conserves energy so your body can better fight off infection and disease. Studies show that people who sleep fewer than six hours a night are more likely to develop a bad cold than people who sleep seven or more hours nightly. And a recent study found that sleep makes vaccines more effective, too.

• **Repairing your body.** Sleep really does restore. The muscles you've challenged during your workouts rebuild and grow while you're asleep, your organs grow new cells, and wounds heal.

• **Boosting your beauty.** Beauty sleep is real. Sleep reduces dark circles and puffiness around your eyes and rehydrates your skin. Plus the growth hormones released while you're asleep help strengthen the collagen structure in your skin cells.

Early to Bed and Early to Rise

A 2012 study in the American Psychological Association journal *Emotion* found that people who get up earlier are more cheerful than night owls. A separate study in the *Journal of Applied Psychology* suggested that morning people tend to be more proactive in many aspects of their lives than late sleepers, which is corroborated by yet another study—in the *Journal of General Psychology*—that found that adults who stay up late also tend to procrastinate more often. In fact, there's a plethora of scientific evidence showing that people who get up earlier maintain a healthier weight, get more exercise, smoke and drink less, and have sunnier dispositions. As for wealthier, well ... health is wealth, right? So set that alarm!

- **Sharpening your mind.** In the United States, more than 70,000 car crashes a year are blamed on sleep deprivation, and lack of sleep has been shown to impair overall reaction time at least as much as being drunk. And it doesn't take long: Just one night of subpar shut-eye can cause a measurable decline in your decision making and judgment, not to mention your reaction time. Adequate sleep is necessary to help learn new information, too.

- **Improving your mood.** Lack of sleep can make you irritable and cranky, which makes you more susceptible to stress and stress-related health problems. That may be unpleasant enough for you, but think about all the people who have to deal with your crabbiness. No wonder people who get enough sleep have better overall dispositions and healthier relationships than those who don't.

- **Calming the chaos.** Our brain has the thankless task of sorting through all the facts, figures, and sensory stimulation that bombard us daily. While we sleep, our brains work on prioritizing, archiving, and cataloging these experiences so that we can retrieve what we need when we need it.

- **Creating happy memories.** Seminal research conducted in 2006 by sleep experts Robert Stickgold and Matthew P. Walker shows that the ability to remember positive words and events deteriorates by 50 percent for those who are sleep-deprived, whereas the recall of negative words and memories lessens by only 20 percent. What does this mean? Inadequate sleep leaves us with more than twice as many negative memories as positive ones, affecting our overall outlook and potentially increasing our risk for depression and other psychiatric disorders.

- **Helping your heart.** This is a big one. Research shows a clear link between sleeping fewer than six hours a night and an increased risk of heart disease. Inadequate sleep doesn't cause heart issues per se, but it adds to the risk factors, including increased inflammation and higher blood pressure. However, adequate sleep reduces inflammation and lowers blood pressure. Win-win.

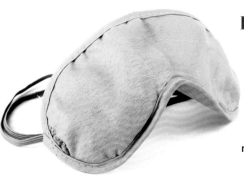

How Does This Magical "Sleep" Thing Work Anyway?

Although most of us don't remember much about our nights except for our very weirdest dreams, there are actually well-defined stages of sleep, which we cycle through three to five times a night. Each full cycle normally lasts between 90 minutes and two hours.

> ## *"Early to bed and early to rise, makes a man healthy, wealthy, and wise."*
>
> —BENJAMIN FRANKLIN

THE STAGES OF SLEEP

Stage 1: Transitional. The shift from wakefulness to light sleep usually lasts about five minutes, during which your muscles begin to relax, your body temperature drops, and your brain activity begins to slow down.

Stage 2: Almost there. This is the first stage of real sleep, lasting anywhere from 10 to 30 minutes. Your heart rate and breathing slow down, although you can still be roused quickly by noise or light.

Stage 3: Now you're talking. This is deep, restorative sleep. Your breathing becomes very slow and regular, your blood pressure falls, your brain waves slow, and your heart rate drops to about 30 percent below normal. It's during

The Magic of Melatonin

The hormone melatonin plays several important roles in your body, including helping to maintain your circadian rhythm (that internal system that tells you when to wake up and when to go to sleep). Melatonin naturally rises when the lights go down (triggering sleep) and falls when things get bright (time to rise). However, melatonin production may drop as we age, which may be one reason sleep quality often deteriorates after we hit 45 or 50.

You can, of course, purchase melatonin supplements at any drugstore, but while supplements have been shown to reduce jet lag for travelers and can help with short-term sleep problems, using them regularly may lead to daytime drowsiness and other issues. For a long-term solution, it's better to boost your own melatonin production by maintaining a consistent bedtime routine and keeping the bedroom cool, dark, and quiet.

this stage that your immune system really kicks into gear and other body systems repair themselves. We spend about 20 percent of our total sleep time in deep sleep, but that percentage starts to decline after age 65.

Stage 4: REM (rapid eye movement). This is, literally, where are dreams are made. Scientists believe the dream stage serves several functions, including increasing our ability to learn and retain information. We generally start with short spurts of REM early in the night, which increase in length toward morning, when it may last for up to 30 minutes. During REM, our body puts most of our muscles into a state of paralysis, presumably so we won't hurt ourselves trying to act out our dreams.

Countdown to Relaxation

Many deep breathing or meditation techniques are likely to help you get to sleep, but one especially easy way to relax is the 4-7-8 breathing method popularized by Andrew Weil. Here's how to do it:

• Place the tip of your tongue on the front ridge of your gum behind your top teeth, and keep it there.
• Breathe in deeply through your nose for four seconds.
• Hold your breath for seven seconds.
• Exhale with a big whooshing sound through your mouth for eight seconds.
• Repeat several times until you're ready to drift off to sleep.

Stage 5: Waking. We wake in the morning, of course, but also intermittently during the night before sinking back into sleep. During waking, our heart and breathing rates increase and our mind becomes more alert. Unfortunately, as we age, the periods of overnight waking may get longer while our sleep duration gets proportionately shorter.

Although the stages are numbered, we tend to weave back and forth between them rather than progressing in order. As a rule, most of us get the majority of our deepest sleep earlier in the night and more of our REM sleep later in the night. However, age and health problems can disrupt our personal sleep pattern.

The Skinny on Sleep Deprivation

More of us are sleeping less. In 2013 only 59 percent of Americans got seven or more hours of sleep a night, which was way down from 1942, when 84 percent did (no Internet back then, you know).

Sleep shortage is a serious problem. About 40 percent of adults report falling asleep unintentionally at least once a month due to lack of shut-eye And many of our major health concerns, including heart disease, diabetes, and obesity, have been linked to lack of sleep.

Popping pills is not the answer. In 2014 alone, more than 42 million sleep-aid prescriptions were filled in the United States However, most sleeping pills are addictive and may disrupt your normal sleep patterns, which is why medical experts say they should be used only as a short-term measure. The long-term solution? Find and fix the cause of your sleep problems. Keep these two tried-and-true principles in mind:

> **Your internal clock rules.** Whether you're a morning lark or a night owl, your circadian rhythm—the internal sense of when to sleep and when to wake—is set during the first few months of life and is very hard to change. We tend to sleep best when we stay in sync with our internal clock and less well when we try to fight it.

> **Exercise improves sleep.** Studies have consistently found the more exercise you get during the day, the better you'll sleep at night—at any age. Regular exercise can help you fall asleep faster and feel more alert during the day. Even a 10-minute walk can improve the duration and quality of your sleep— but people who regularly get vigorous exercise sleep best of all.

Wait...Do We Really Need More Sleep?

A study published in 2015 in *Current Biology,* tracked the sleep habits of three hunter-gatherer tribes in Africa and South America. It found that in these nonindustrialized societies (read: no lights or electronics), people sleep about six and a half hours per night, which is even less than the average American. While some experts took this to mean we don't need as much sleep as has been recommended, others say the study didn't account for differences in the *quality* of sleep, including the fact that insomnia is experienced far less in the tribes studied. One interesting theory suggests that the total time period of sleep may be less important than the ambient temperature, since all the hunter-gatherers slept when the night was coolest and woke after the air began to warm.

Could You Have a Sleep Disorder?

As many as 70 million Americans suffer from at least one chronic sleep disorder—a definite downer in our quest to stay well rested. Serious as they can be, many sleep disorders have a simple solution. But left untreated, they can get even worse, leading to mood swings, anxiety, and depression, as well as memory problems, difficulty thinking clearly, and serious accidents.

The most common sleep disorders are:

INSOMNIA. A pronounced difficulty getting to sleep or staying asleep, which can be either short-term or chronic and may come and go over time.
Watch for: Lying awake for more than 30 minutes after going to bed; waking often during the night; taking a long time to get back to sleep once awake; waking up too early in the morning and not being able to get back to sleep.
Risk factors: Can be triggered or worsened by poor diet, stress, anxiety, depression, frequent changes in bedtime or work schedule, lack of exercise, and poor sleep habits. Medical conditions, like overactive thyroid, heartburn, and breathing disorders, can cause insomnia, as can alcohol, tobacco, and certain medications.

SLEEP APNEA. A potentially dangerous condition in which the air passages become restricted during sleep to the extent that a person may temporarily stop breathing.
Watch for: Loud snoring—especially if it includes pauses followed by gasping or choking, dry mouth or sore throat in the morning, and morning headaches. Sleep apnea can be treated through methods including changing sleep habits and using special pillows or custom mouthpieces. Severe cases may need a breathing device called a CPAP, or even surgery.
Risk factors: Sleep apnea is a common symptom of obesity, but people of all sizes can be affected, especially if they have congenitally small airways, or if their airways are swollen due to allergy or illness. It tends to be worsened by sleeping on the back.

RESTLESS LEGS SYNDROME (RLS). A neurological disorder characterized by tingling, burning, or other sensations that make you want to move your legs when you're resting. RLS affects as many as 10 percent of adults and is more common among women than men. It may be inherited or may be triggered by another illness, in which case treating the underlying condition may reduce RLS.
Watch for: A strong urge to move your legs and aching or unpleasant sensations, especially in the calves. The feeling gets worse in the evening and when you are inactive or resting,

and improves if you move or rub your legs. In chronic cases, it can be managed with life-style changes, exercise, relaxation techniques, massage, and medication.

Risk factors: Genetics, iron deficiency, pregnancy, kidney disease, Parkinson's disease, diabetes, rheumatoid arthritis, or nerve damage. Some medications, including certain antidepressants, allergy medications, and drugs used to treat heart disease or high blood pressure may contribute to RLS.

PARASOMNIA. An umbrella term for a group of several different sleep disorders including sleepwalking, sleep terrors, sleep paralysis, and other abnormal sleep behaviors that affect up to 4 percent of adults. In addition to losing sleep, parasomniacs can seriously injure themselves or others during these episodes.

Watch for: Partners and family members are often the first to spot parasomniac behavior, but symptoms include nightmares, a feeling of paralysis when falling asleep or waking up, and teeth grinding during sleep. Most parasomniacs can be treated with better sleep habits or by addressing the underlying cause.

Risk factors: Genetics, sleep apnea, and certain brain disorders may predispose people to parasomnia, but it can also be triggered by traumatic events, depression, poor sleep habits, and certain medications, including common prescription and over-the-counter sleep aids.

NARCOLEPSY. A disorder marked by interrupted sleep, falling asleep at inappropriate times, sleep paralysis, sudden muscle weakness, and hallucinations when falling asleep.

Watch for: Short, intense periods of sleepiness during the day, possibly triggered by strong emotions; falling asleep suddenly and unintentionally during the day; sudden muscle weakness in one part of your body; a feeling of paralysis while falling asleep or waking up. Narcolepsy cannot be cured but can be managed with medication and other options.

Risk factors: Narcolepsy may be triggered by a combination of factors, including genetics, brain injuries, infections, autoimmune disorders, or toxin exposure.

SEE A DOCTOR IF YOU HAVE ANY OF THE ABOVE SYMPTOMS OR IF YOU:

- Yawn, blink a lot, or feel excessively drowsy during the day despite getting adequate hours of sleep
- Have trouble focusing on your tasks
- Frequently feel irritable and have trouble regulating your mood
- Experience unexplained weight gain or loss
- Snore or twitch a lot in your sleep
- Sweat a lot while you sleep—and aren't going through menopause
- Have unexplained muscle aches

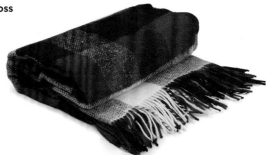

Come, Sleep! O Sleep, the certain knot of peace ..."

—SIR PHILIP SIDNEY

Sleep Aids: With Friends Like These, Who Needs Enemies?

Oh, yes. When sleep gets hard to find, I absolutely understand the temptation to swing by the drugstore in search of a chemical snooze-generator. But relying on prescription or even over-the-counter (OTC) sleep aids for more than a couple of weeks is a very bad idea that can lead to larger problems.

A PRESCRIPTION FOR TROUBLE

Most drugs intended to lull you to sleep are literally lulling you. Prescription options like Lunesta and Ambien are in a class of medication known as sedative hypnotics, and they come with a slew of unintended consequences.

You may remember the headlines from the early 2000s about Ambien, one of the most popular sleep aids of all time. For several years, there were regular reports about Ambien users who went to bed and later woke up to discover that they'd been walking, talking, eating, and, worst of all, driving and causing car accidents—all without

Snacks to Sleep On

A light snack eaten about an hour before bed may improve sleep by triggering relaxation hormones, like serotonin, and creating a quick rise and fall in blood-sugar levels. Foods like nuts, seeds, and honey, for instance, contain tryptophan, the famously sedating amino acid found in turkey. But choose mild foods and keep the portions small, or you may find yourself dreaming of antacids.

Nibble these for a good night:
Walnuts, almonds, cheese and crackers, oatmeal, warm milk with honey, rice, popcorn, chamomile tea, or passion-fruit tea

Want to stay awake? Try these:
Coffee, black tea, other caffeinated beverages, soda, fried foods, fatty foods, spicy foods, chocolate, or sugary desserts

having any memory of their overnight misadventures. And the dangerous behavior didn't stop in the morning. Many people who used Ambien to sleep at night ended up having such severe drowsiness the next day that they caused hundreds of additional car accidents—some of them fatal.

In 2013 the FDA finally ordered doctors to halve the recommended doses of Ambien and similar drugs, due to these concerns. But even in smaller amounts, these drugs can disrupt your sleep patterns, impair your daytime alertness, and increase your risk of falls and accidents. And, of course, there's the little matter of addiction: Sedative hypnotics tend to be habit-forming, which means that if you start relying on them to fall asleep, they'll make it hard for you to fall asleep without them. *Anti-bonus:* The side effects hit women even harder than men, because it takes us longer to metabolize these drugs.

The Sweet Smell of Sleep

Aromatherapy can be effective for inducing sleep. Add a sachet to your pillow, or sprinkle a few drops of essential oils into a diffuser or onto a handkerchief that you can tuck into your pillowcase. As to which aroma works best, lavender's impressive sedative effects are well documented, but vetiver, chamomile, jasmine, and vanilla are among the other scents that have been shown to improve sleep.

LEAVE OTCS ON THE COUNTER
If you're thinking that OTC options are a better choice, think again. Most OTC sleep aids rely on antihistamines, which can leave you feeling hungover in the morning and may have other side effects, including triggering dangerous drug interactions and certain medical conditions. If you've ever tried using certain allergy medications as a sleep aid, you're essentially doing the same thing. What's more, your body adapts to antihistamine-based sleep aids quickly, meaning you'd have to keep upping the dose to get the same results.

THE DIRTY LITTLE SECRET OF SLEEP AIDS
They may help you get to sleep a few minutes faster—although even that's debatable—but most of them don't really help you sleep any better and may leave you feeling drowsy the next day, creating an endless chain of exhaustion.

TAKE BACK YOUR NIGHT WITH BETTER SLEEP HYGIENE
Better bet? There's a simple, effective, and totally side-effect-free treatment that has been shown to improve sleep for three-quarters of people who've tried it and to completely eliminate insomnia for at least half of them. Known by such totally unsexy

names as "behavioral treatment intervention" and "sleep hygiene education," the concept is that you can cure insomnia simply by practicing these good sleep habits:

- Go to bed when you're tired.

- Restrict the time you spend sleeping to the minimum you need to feel rested.

- Get up at a consistent time.

- Don't stay in bed if you aren't sleeping.

Accompanied by basic relaxation techniques and—only if needed—nonpharmaceutical light therapy to help reset an out-of-balance biological clock, simply adopting these four habits is all most of us need to kick the insomnia monkey off our back—without letting a new monkey climb on.

Positioned for Success

Sleep apnea, snoring, headaches, neck and back pain, and heartburn can all be aggravated by a less-than-ideal sleep posture. If you wake up feeling worse than when you lay down, consider changing how you spend your nights. And choose pillows that support you properly with these tips:

ON YOUR BACK

- *Pros:* For most of us, this is probably the best position. It preserves a normal alignment for your neck and back, reduces acid reflux, and helps prevent unwanted wrinkles, because your face isn't touching the pillow.

- *Cons:* Because the base of the tongue falls back across the airway, back sleepers snore more and may be at higher risk for sleep apnea.

- *Pillow talk:* Choose a medium pillow to support your head just enough that your neck stays in a natural curve. Try a small bolster or rolled towel under your knees to keep your hips relaxed.

ON YOUR SIDE

- *Pros:* Snoring is reduced compared to back sleeping. The spine is elongated, so back pain may be relieved, and sleeping on your left side may help to reduce acid reflux and heartburn.

> ## " *Sleep is the golden chain that binds health and our bodies together.*"
>
> —THOMAS DEKKER

- *Cons:* Side sleepers are more prone to wrinkles, since their face is squashed into the pillow. Arms will have restricted blood flow, which can lead to circulation problems, and neck and shoulder problems may be exacerbated.

- *Pillow talk:* Choose a firm pillow that keeps your head in line with the rest of your spine. Add a thin pillow between your knees to reduce spinal twisting. And if heartburn or acid reflux is a problem, try a thin or wedge-shaped pillow to elevate your shoulders slightly.

ON YOUR STOMACH

- *Pros:* Reduces the likelihood of snoring or sleep apnea.

- *Cons:* Sorry, stomach snoozers! This is generally the worst way to sleep. This position flattens the natural curve of your back, which may cause low-back pain, and puts unnecessary pressure on the neck and joints. And, of course, it scrunches up your face, adding to wrinkles.

- *Pillow talk:* If you must sleep on your stomach, avoid kinking your neck more than necessary: Choose a thin, soft pillow or none at all.

Sleep Your Way to the Top

If sleep isn't a fountain of youth, it's certainly a built-in rejuvenator and a cornerstone of long-term health. But how much do we need and—perhaps a better question—how the heck are we supposed to get it?

HOW MUCH IS ENOUGH?

The evidence on this is pretty conclusive. The National Sleep Foundation recommends that everyone between the ages of 26 and 64 should aim for seven to nine hours of sleep every night, and people 65 and over should get seven to eight hours. That's still a big range, so allow your body to dictate your personal requirement. Go to bed early enough that you could sleep at least seven hours if you wanted to. If you're bright-eyed at 5 a.m., that's great. (But don't wake me when you get up, okay?)

Sweet Dreams

Luckily, we live in an age where myriad tools are at our disposal specifically designed to help us drift off into a dreamy slumber. Fluffy down pillows, mattresses that allow us to adjust temperatures and positions, noise machines that block out sounds that can keep us awake, amber-emitting lamps, and headbands that induce sleep through sound waves are just a few of the gadgets that can help the effort.

Whether it's by technology or counting sheep, getting a good night's sleep is as important as daily exercise, eating well, and managing stress. Experts now understand that adequate sleep does much more for our overall health and well-being than we ever imagined. Sleep helps keep our brains sharp and bodies healthy, and it brightens our moods.

10 Small Steps to Sound Rest

❶ In the morning: Make your bed—it will feel more soothing when you get into it tonight. And get some exercise.

❷ All day long: Eat well and stay active.

❸ 8 hours before bedtime: Cut off the caffeine.

❹ 4 hours before bedtime: No more alcohol.

❺ 2 hours before bedtime: Take a warm bath or shower.

❻ 90 minutes before bedtime: Turn off the TV and computer, and put away your phone and other electron-

ics. Make a list of anything you need to do tomorrow, then forget about it.

❼ 1 hour before bedtime: Last call for a bedtime snack (a snack, not a meal!). Put away the water glass. Start dimming the lights.

❽ 30 minutes before bedtime: Wash your face, brush your teeth, and wrap up your personal routine.

❾ 15 minutes before bed: Do a few minutes of meditation or relaxation exercises.

❿ 1 minute before bed: Put on socks—warm feet help you fall asleep faster.

A Good Night's Sleep

If you're in the dark about how to actually get enough sleep, start implementing these effective strategies to clean up your sleep hygiene.

INSTEAD OF MAKING YOUR BEDROOM COMMAND CENTRAL,

Reserve the master suite for S&S. Stick to only two activities in your bedroom: sleep and sex. If your bedroom also serves as an office, TV room, and social media hub, your brain will associate it with higher levels of stimulation and you'll have a harder time winding down.

INSTEAD OF WATCHING TV ALL EVENING,

Turn off the tube at least 90 minutes before bed. Exciting entertainment, especially action-packed or violent imagery, can wind you up and keep you from falling asleep. Restrict television to the early evening, choose stress-releasing comedies over adrenaline-raising thrillers, and keep screens out of the bedroom completely.

INSTEAD OF PILLOW TALK WITH YOUR FACEBOOK FRIENDS,

Make your bedroom a no-Internet zone. Not only will surfing the web and updating your status stimulate instead of calm you, the "blue" lights emitted from many smartphones, tablets, and computers suppress melatonin production, interfering with your ability to get to sleep. Even if your device is equipped with a nighttime mode, it's still keeping your brain away from snooze mode.

INSTEAD OF KEEPING THE NIGHT-LIGHT BURNING,

Put the lights out. Our brains interpret light as a cue for wakefulness, and light can suppress your body's production of melatonin, the primary hormone for triggering sleep. Darkness, on the other hand, tells your brain it's time for sleep. If you need to find your way to the bathroom, try a motion-activated night-light. And if you must leave the lights on for someone else, channel your inner Holly Golightly and wear a sleep mask, or look into "sleep lights," designed to enhance rest.

INSTEAD OF TOSSING AND TURNING FOR HOURS,

Get back up. Most of us fall asleep in about 10 minutes. If you're still awake after 30, then get out of bed for a while. Otherwise you risk getting so stressed about not sleeping that you condition your brain to associate "bed" with "can't sleep." Keep the lights dim and go into another room to meditate, stretch, read, or do some other low-key activity until you feel drowsy and relaxed. (No TV or digital devices, though!) Then slide back into bed and go to sleep.

INSTEAD OF SUFFERING THROUGH THE SNORING,

Shut down the chain saw. Snoring is very common, especially as we age, but whether you or your bedmate is the culprit (for what it's worth, men are statistically more likely to snore), the noise can ruin your slumber and may indicate sleep apnea. For garden-variety snoring, try nasal strips to help open up nasal passages for quieter sleep, or use earplugs. Back sleepers tend to snore most often, so if it's you, try sleeping on your side—and if it isn't, gently nudge your partner to roll over. Still, if it happens often enough to interfere with sleep, talk with a doctor about possible causes. Most of the time, it's fixable.

INSTEAD OF DRINKING COFFEE ALL DAY,

Ban caffeine after 2 p.m. Caffeine keeps you awake not only by acting as a stimulant, but also by blocking adenosine, a brain chemical that helps you fall asleep. The effects from caffeinated drinks and foods can linger in your system many hours after you consume them, so restrict them to the first half of your day.

INSTEAD OF POURING A NIGHTCAP,

Have your last drink at least four hours before you go to bed. Sure, alcohol will make you feel drowsy for a while. But it will also disrupt your sleep pattern, likely waking you up long before dawn. It also reduces critical REM sleep and can make you urinate more frequently.

INSTEAD OF DRINKING WATER LATE AT NIGHT,

Stop sipping at least an hour before bed. Hydration is important, but waking up in the middle of the night to go to the bathroom really cuts into sleep. If you find yourself doing it often, don't exacerbate the problem by drinking more. However, if you wake up in the wee hours because you're parched from dry mouth or panting from night sweats, it might be worth keeping a small glass by your bed for a sip or two.

INSTEAD OF SMOKING TO RELAX,

Stop smoking already! Better shut-eye is just one of the thousands of reasons to quit. Among the many proven dangers of cigarettes, nicotine—a stimulant, not a relaxant—can wreck your slumber. (As well as your heart and lungs and skin and bones and teeth and ...)

INSTEAD OF EXERCISING AT NIGHT,

Work out early in the day. The benefits of daily aerobic exercise include the trifecta of good sleep: get to sleep faster; spend more time in deep sleep; and wake up less frequently during the night. But if you work out close to bedtime, you may be too energized to reap the rewards. If evening is your only option, opt for a relaxing walk or yoga session rather than high-powered or competitive activities, which can boost your adrenaline levels and keep you awake.

INSTEAD OF FRETTING OVER TOMORROW'S TO-DO LIST,

Write it down. Many people who suffer from insomnia say they can't sleep because they're worried about all the things they have to do. But there's evidence that simply putting your thoughts in writing by journaling or making a task list will help lower your stress levels and relax your mind.

INSTEAD OF TAKING YOUR STRESS TO BED,

Meditate before you lie down. A few minutes of deep breathing and meditation help settle the brain's arousal system and release sleep-disrupting stress, preparing you for a good night's sleep.

INSTEAD OF CRANKING THE HEAT TO GET COZY,

Keep it cool. Keeping the temperature between 60 and 67 degrees causes our body temperatures to drop as well, which helps us to transition to sleep more quickly and stay asleep longer. You can boost that effect by taking a warm bath or shower an hour or two before bed. Your body will compensate by lowering your internal temperature just in time to send you to dreamland.

INSTEAD OF SAYING, "NOT TONIGHT. I'M TOO TIRED,"

Use sex to wind down. Sex is a fantastic (and all-natural!) relaxant, and the hormones released during and after sex can promote a good night's sleep. And, in a sweet bit of positive reinforcement, getting better sleep tonight will help you feel even sexier tomorrow.

INSTEAD OF SLEEPING IN ON WEEKENDS,

Stick to a regular schedule. While I dream of lounging until noon on my (imaginary) days off, the National Sleep Foundation says it's actually a terrible idea. It won't result in restful slumber and will disrupt your internal clock even further. A consistent routine (same time to bed, same time to rise) of adequate sleep will provide the maximum benefits of sleep and reduce the risk of insomnia.

INSTEAD OF FEELING GROGGY IN THE AFTERNOON,

Take a short siesta. If you're getting as much nighttime sleep as possible but you still feel tired midday, take a 20-minute nap. Right after lunch is ideal, since you'll have a full tummy to help relax you and it's not too close to bedtime. Just be careful not to snooze too long or you'll risk disrupting your critical nighttime sleep.

INSTEAD OF WORRYING THAT YOU'RE MISSING OUT ON LIFE BY SLEEPING,

Think about how much more of life you'll enjoy when you're awake. Sure, you might have to record *The Late Show* for tomorrow evening, but if you go to bed earlier and sleep longer, you'll start the day in a better mood—and get more out of it, too. And, yes, you ought to say no to a glass of wine at 10 p.m., but you can really enjoy the one you pour at 6. It's all about prioritizing. And the highest priority is your quality of life.

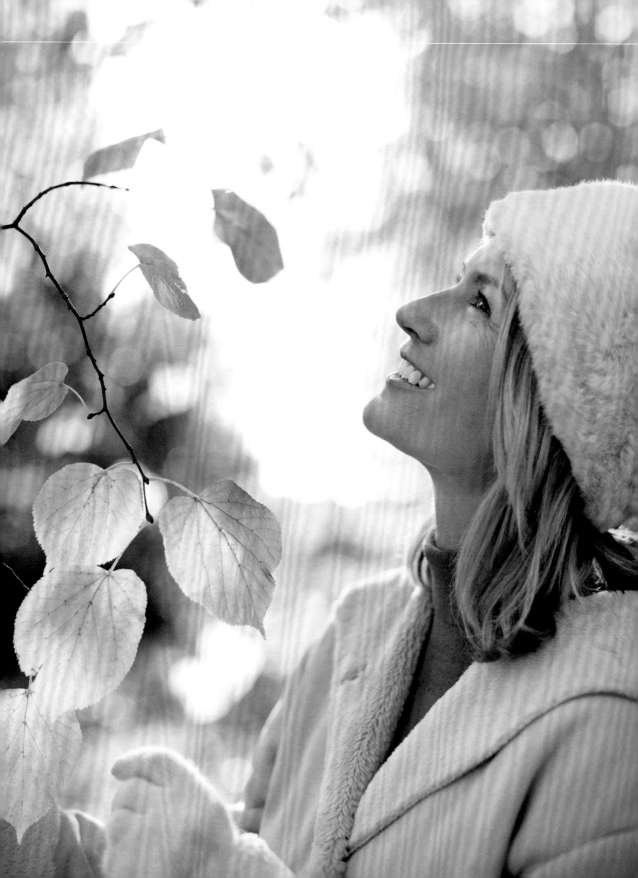

CHAPTER 5

Menopause, the Magical Mystery Tour

"There is no more creative force in the world than the menopausal woman with zest."

—MARGARET MEAD

Ah, yes. Now things get really exciting. Maybe you've already gone through "the change"—a quaint little euphemism from days of yore. Or maybe you're in the throes of it right now. But if you're not yet at the point when estrogen levels start going down, down, down, you might want to heed the words of Bette Davis in *All About Eve:* "Fasten your seat belts. It's going to be a bumpy night."

Except it's far more than a night. It's years. Several years, in fact …

How long?!?

Yep, it's true. Perimenopause—the transition to menopause—usually starts in your 40s or even earlier, but according to the North American Menopause Society (NAMS), the average woman doesn't actually reach menopause until age 51.

Ready for some good news? Once you hit menopause, you are then, officially, a postmenopausal woman—for the rest of your life. And since most women born after 1950 will live well into their 80s or beyond, that means almost half of your life will probably be spent as a postmenopausal woman.

And here's some even better news: While menopause often causes some uncomfortable (but temporary!) symptoms, the majority of women do not experience major changes in their quality of life during menopause. And afterward, post-menopausal women enjoy a new sense of freedom and relief. Do we miss our periods? No. Are we happy to have sex without worrying about getting pregnant? Yes! And the truth is that most of us make it through the whole process with only a few rough spots along the way.

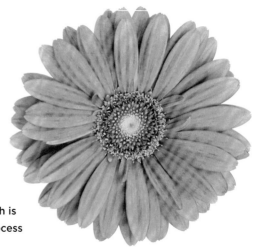

Estrogen: The Reason for the Mayhem

Whichever stage of menopause you're in, estrogen (and, to a lesser degree, its BFF progesterone) is probably rocking your world.

Estrogen hormones have many functions in our bodies, but their biggest responsibility is controlling reproductive health, so as we age out of prime pregnancy years, estrogen levels start to fluctuate, initiating perimenopause. And when we get to menopause itself? Estrogen goes into free fall. When we come out the other side—and we all do—our estrogen levels are significantly lower than when we started.

The Stages of Menopause

Although it's common to refer to the entire menopausal transition simply as "menopause," it's helpful to break it down into stages to better understand what's going on in your body along the way.

PERIMENOPAUSE

> What's happening: Your body begins to produce less estrogen as your child-bearing years wind down.

> Major symptoms: Menstrual periods are irregular, becoming lighter or heavier, longer or shorter, and more or less frequent, until you start skipping some. Pregnancy is still possible, but it may become harder to conceive and the likelihood of complications increases. Other conspicuous symptoms include hot flashes, night sweats, and mood swings.

Starts: In your 40s, but earlier is possible.

Lasts: Anywhere from two to 15 years, but four to five years is average. Symptoms may become more pronounced as you get closer to menopause.

MENOPAUSE

What's happening: Technically menopause is when you stop ovulating and can no longer get pregnant. However, it's pretty hard to pinpoint that moment, because cycles can get erratic during perimenopause. The proof is when you've gone a full year without a period. In the two or three years on either side of that transition, estrogen falls dramatically, which can trigger an array of secondary issues.

Major symptoms: Hot flashes, night sweats, and mood swings are the biggies, but other signs may include vaginal dryness, dry skin and eyes, decreased sex drive, increased breast tenderness, difficulty sleeping, forgetfulness, and weight gain.

Starts: On average, women reach menopause around age 51.

Lasts: You're through menopause when you've gone a full year without having a menstrual period. And if you have one after 11 months? Start the clock over again.

POSTMENOPAUSE

What's happening: Estrogen levels stabilize at their new, lower levels.

Major symptoms: The good: You're done with periods, and the major symptoms of the menopausal

Menopause Is Universal, but Also Personal

• In 1998 there were over 477 million postmenopausal women worldwide. By 2025, that number will be over 1.1 billion.
• Genetics plays a very strong role in determining your personal menopause time frame.
• Black women experience menopausal symptoms like hot flashes about four years longer than their Caucasian girlfriends and two years longer than Hispanic women.
• Women who smoke may reach menopause one to two years earlier than nonsmokers.
• Some women start having hot flashes even before perimenopause begins.
• More than 75 percent of all women experience some symptoms of menopause, but only a small percentage are debilitated by them.

MENOPAUSE, THE MAGICAL MYSTERY TOUR

"*Nothing is so painful to the human mind as a great and sudden change.*"

—MARY SHELLEY

transition fade away. The not-so-good: Lower estrogen can lead to lower bone density, muscle loss, and weight gain, as well as head-to-toe dryness. You're also at a higher risk for some medical issues, including urinary incontinence and heart disease.

Starts: As soon as you hit menopause, you're into postmenopause.

Lasts: For the rest of your life.

Making It to the Other Side

I'll admit I was pretty lucky on this one. Menopause handed me a few sleepless nights, a handful of heat waves, a few extra pounds (that I shed eventually), and voilà: I was done. Okay, maybe it wasn't quite that fast. But it wasn't that bad, either. I entered menopause easier than a lot of women.

However, for many women, this transition can be one of the most challenging times of their lives. The hormonal drop can trigger severe physical symptoms, significant weight gain, feelings of depression, fear, and isolation—and more.

So if you're having a hard time of it, listen up, because there are many lifestyle changes and medical options that can make this transition easier. We have hormone replacement therapy, of course, plus we know much more about the ways nutrition, exercise, and other habits can reduce or even eliminate many of the symptoms and health risks of menopause.

The short version? No one in this day and age should suffer needlessly, and that means *you*. So instead of bemoaning your fate, be grateful you're able to embrace the modern-day benefits of being a postmenopausal woman and avail yourself of modern-day help to manage the more challenging aspects of menopause itself.

Introducing TMT:
The Terrible Menopause
Trifecta

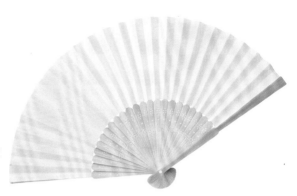

For most women, the most obvious—and problematic—symptoms of menopause are what I call the terrible menopause trifecta (TMT) of hot flashes, night sweats, and mood swings. What are they?

Hot flashes. Technically known as vasomotor symptoms, hot flashes are caused by hormonal fluctuations. Most women experience them as a sudden surge of heat, especially on the face and neck, making you feel flushed and sweaty. Flashes may also be accompanied by a rapid heartbeat, often followed by feeling chilled. Hot flashes may occur only once in a while or as often as several times a day and usually last for two to 30 minutes at a stretch. Their frequency and severity are partly influenced by genetics—which you can't control—but they tend to be much worse for women who smoke, are overweight, or eat a lot of sugar. Hot weather, alcohol, caffeine, and spicy foods can also trigger or worsen hot flashes.

Night sweats. Hot flashes seem to be even more common while we're sleeping, when they're known as night sweats. And they're especially cruel—waking us up and disrupting our sleep cycle at exactly the time in our life when we would benefit from more shut-eye.

Mood swings. While they may sound minor, mood swings can actually be the worst part of menopause as they can affect our friends and family, too. They are primarily caused by fluctuating hormone levels, which affect the way brain chemicals function, leaving us blindsided by rage or sobbing in despair over nothing at all. But mood swings are—obviously—greatly exacerbated by lack of sleep, as well as by poor diet, lack of exercise, external stress, and changing life circumstances, like children leaving home or parents needing help. To make things worse, for many women, mood swings are accompanied by memory problems, like forgetfulness.

No matter how terrible TMT symptoms seem, there is a bright side! They are all easily treatable—and they're all temporary.

Cool It, Sister

I won't lie: Hot flashes are annoying and uncomfortable. But there are several things you can do to make them both less severe and less disruptive.

TAKE A DEEP BREATH. Simple as it sounds, relaxation breathing has been clinically shown to reduce the severity of hot flashes. Take several slow, deep breaths into your belly as soon as you feel the heat rising. For extra cooling power, either stick out your tongue, curl it, and sip in the air like you're drinking through a straw, or place the tip of your tongue behind your upper teeth and breathe in around it. Exhale completely each time.

DRINK SOMETHING COLD. If you feel a hot flash coming on, grab a glass of ice water and start sipping. The more ice, the better.

ICE IT. No, it won't look good in a board meeting, but if the occasion permits, try rubbing an ice cube, ice pack, or even a cold washcloth on the insides of your wrists or back of your neck.

AVOID WARM ROOMS. Even if the temperature seems okay to other people, it might feel like an inferno to you. Either excuse yourself or stake out a seat near an open window or by a fan. Keep the temperature in your house cool.

EAT MORE ISOFLAVONES. Isoflavones are naturally occurring phytoestrogens, which act like a weaker form of estrogen in the body and have been clinically demonstrated to reduce hot flashes. They're found in lentils, ground flaxseed, and chickpeas, but they are most abundant in soy foods, like tofu and tempeh. However, there's been some question about whether phytoestrogens are safe for women who have had breast cancer or are at high risk for it. If that's you, check with your doctor before you supersize your soy milk.

IDENTIFY YOUR TRIGGERS—AND AVOID THEM. Some women find that caffeine, alcohol, or certain foods tend to set off hot flashes. Triggers can be fairly individualized, so if you feel a heat wave rising, think back to everything you ate or drank recently and write it down. If you spot a pattern, change your habits.

DRESS FOR THE WEATHER—INSIDE AND OUT

When hot flashes become part of your life, a little advance planning can make them more manageable without giving up on glamour.

LAYER, LAYER, LAYER. You want to be able to peel off some clothes—and add them back on—and still look appropriate in any situation. Opt for light layers and steer clear of super-tight clothes, which can make things worse. If you start with a sleeveless or short-sleeve base layer, add a lightweight cardigan or jacket, and top it all off with a scarf, you'll be able to adjust throughout the day and still look great.

CHOOSE BREATHABLE FIBERS. Silk, bamboo, and merino wool all wick sweat and help regulate body temperature. Cotton breathes well but doesn't dry quickly if you perspire. If you tend to have a lot of underarm perspiration, try washable dress shields to absorb excess sweat and protect your clothes.

THINK ABOUT FOOTWEAR, TOO. If your feet tend to get hot, stick to lower-cut shoes and booties rather than knee-high boots. Sandals are great, but peep-toe and d'Orsay styles also offer a little ventilation during cooler weather.

WEAR ICY JEWELRY. There are necklaces on the market that you can freeze overnight before wearing to help keep your cool.

IN THE HEAT OF THE NIGHT

Instead of sleeplessly sweating your way through the night, try these tips for cooling off:

KEEP YOUR BEDROOM COOL. Turn off the heat, turn on the AC, or open a window. Whatever you do, get the temp between 60 and 67 for the best chance at a restful night.

FAN YOURSELF. Keep a small electric fan on a table or chair next to your bed, pointed directly at you. An oscillating model will sweep over you from head to toe.

SLEEP WITH SEVERAL LIGHT BEDCOVERS rather than a single heavy comforter so you can adjust layers throughout the night.

DON'T COVER YOUR ENTIRE BODY. Keeping a foot, shoulder, or arm uncovered at night can help your body release extra heat.

LET YOUR BODY BREATHE. Sleeping in the buff has a lot of health benefits, including temperature regulation. But if you don't want to go nude, try shorts and tanks made of wicking fabric, to keep you from getting clammy—and skip the undies underneath. *Tip:* Clothes sold as athletic wear can also make great pj's.

Beyond TMT

As estrogen tanks, it also triggers a cascade of changes that impact nearly every part of our body (take note of how often the word "dry" pops up):

- Skin becomes drier, thinner, less elastic, and weaker.

- Eyes get dry and irritated.

- Hair can dry out, lose luster, and get thinner.

- Sex can become uncomfortable or even painful, due to a decrease in collagen, which causes the walls of the vagina and urethra to become thinner and drier. This loss of collagen sometimes also leads to incontinence and bladder leaks.

- Bones lose density, putting us at greater risk for fractures and osteoporosis.

- Our metabolism slows, leading to gain weight, especially around the abdomen, which can add to the risk of type 2 diabetes and other health issues.

- We lose muscle tone and may suffer more muscle and joint pain.

- Our cholesterol balance can shift, increasing our risk of heart disease.

- An overstimulation of the nervous and circulatory systems can trigger irregular heartbeats and palpitations.

- Gums can bleed more often.

But don't sweat it! Every single one of these changes in your body can be addressed. Tackle them head-on and your life will be better, now and forevermore.

How to Calm the Chaos

Whatever degree of discomfort you have, there are things you can do to cope with the symptoms of menopause. The best strategy is to think about your short game and your long game at the same time.

Short-term: Address the temporary symptoms of menopause as soon as they crop up.

Long-term: Protect your body from the negative health effects of reduced estrogen.

Bonus: Many of the options at your disposal will do both!

Bring Out the Big Guns:
Hormone Replacement Therapy

One of the biggest—and most controversial—advances in managing menopause over the past few decades has been hormone replacement therapy (HRT), which uses low doses of synthetic hormones to compensate for the loss of estrogen and alleviate the most common symptoms of menopause, including hot flashes, mood swings, and bone loss. HRT has been shown to be highly effective in easing the menopausal transition, but several clinical studies in recent years have shown that it does not protect against memory loss as was once believed and can slightly increase the risk of breast cancer, uterine cancer, heart disease, and stroke, although these risks go back down once treatment is stopped.

Based on the current evidence, however, both the North American Menopause Society and the Endocrine Society agree that HRT can be the right treatment to address temporary symptoms for many otherwise healthy women. While HRT should not be used to treat chronic illnesses and should be prescribed only after your doctor has factored in your health risks and family history of cancer, it can offer welcome relief to many women who are experiencing the most debilitating symptoms of menopause.

HRT is usually prescribed as a combination of both estrogen and progesterone in order to protect against an elevated risk of uterine cancer, but women who have had hysterectomies may be able to take estrogen only. It is available in several forms, ranging from pills to a patch, gel, or spray that allows the hormones to be absorbed through the skin. If you decide to give it a try, work with your gynecologist or PCP to find the lowest dose that alleviates your symptoms, and be sure to reevaluate your treatment plan every six months.

WONDERING IF HRT IS RIGHT FOR YOU?
Ask an expert. Discuss your personal needs and health history with your PCP or ob-gyn, and get the most up-to-date information about HRT.

ABOUT BIOIDENTICAL HORMONE THERAPY ...
In the past several years, another option has been marketed to women concerned about the possible side effects of HRT. Bioidentical hormones are substances that are chemically identical to the hormones we make in our bodies. They are based on plant extracts but are created in laboratories and typically sold through compounding pharmacies that mix the

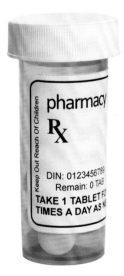

hormones with other substances to create a pill, patch, or cream for patients.

- **What's the problem with bioidentical hormones?** Some bioidentical hormones have been approved by the FDA and may be prescribed by physicians for women who have an allergy or other reaction to conventional HRT. But many others, which have not been tested or approved for safety or efficacy, are being falsely advertised by pharmacies and other companies as "more natural" or "safer" than conventional HRT. Some even claim to be customized based on the hormones in your saliva, which is misleading, because you can't reliably measure hormone levels in your body from saliva.

- **Are they safe?** Contrary to the advertising claims, bioidentical hormones have the same risks as conventional HRT and might actually pose additional problems, especially if they are not FDA-approved. Unapproved drugs haven't been tested to ensure that they release appropriate doses, for instance, so they could increase the risk of uterine cancer and other health issues.

- **How many women use bioidentical hormones?** According to NAMS, 34 percent of menopausal women who take replacement hormones are now using bioidentical hormones, and that percentage is likely to rise, largely because recent hype from celebrities—rather than medical professionals—has led younger women to believe that these supposedly plant-based chemicals are somehow better than conventional HRT. Do your own research.

- **Is it right for me?** If your symptoms are severe, talk with your doctor about HRT. If HRT is not an option, discuss other therapies with your doc, including bioidentical hormones. But never trust your health to marketing propaganda.

There Are Nonhormonal Options, Too

Several prescription medications other than HRT are available to help reduce temporary menopause symptoms, like hot flashes and mood swings. Talk to your doctor to figure out if any of these alternative treatments are right for you:

- **Low-dose mesylate salt of paroxetine (LDMP)** is the only nonhormonal treatment that is FDA-approved for menopausal symptoms. Although paroxetine was originally developed as an antidepressant, a dose of 7.5 mg per day has been proved to reduce both the severity and frequency of hot flashes.

- **Other low-dose antidepressants,** including certain selective serotonin reuptake inhibitors (SSRIs), like escitalopram, and serotonin-norepinephrine reuptake inhibitors (SNRIs), like venlafaxine, have been shown to alleviate hot flashes as well as regulate mood. None are FDA-approved for this purpose yet, but physicians may be able to prescribe them as an off-label treatment option.

- **Gabapentin** is an epilepsy drug that has also been shown to reduce hot flashes and may be prescribed as an off-label treatment option.

What Else Can You Do?

Anything that promotes overall health will help ease you through the menopausal transition more comfortably, because when your body is working well, it can adapt to changes more smoothly and with fewer side effects. Smoking, stress, exhaustion, poor diet, and lack of physical activity will all worsen whatever symptoms you have, so set yourself up for success by practicing excellent self-care. In particular, try to incorporate these healthy habits:

- **Vigorous exercise** that makes you sweat and pant, for around 45 minutes at a stretch, has been shown to significantly reduce hot flashes and night sweats. Even moderate exercise, like walking briskly, can help reduce mood swings, depression, and anxiety by releasing endorphins and other mood-boosting hormones. And, of course, exercise helps you lose weight, which can also help reduce the frequency and severity of hot flashes.

- **A Mediterranean-style diet** that centers on vegetables, fruits, and whole grains has been proved to diminish hot flashes and other menopausal symptoms, whereas a diet heavy on fats and sugars makes them worse. A healthy diet also heads off all those unwanted menopausal pounds.

- **Massage,** especially aromatherapy massage, has been shown to help with hot flashes. Researchers haven't pinpointed why it works, but many women find that reducing stress and anxiety—which massage is known to do very well—helps to squash many menopausal symptoms.

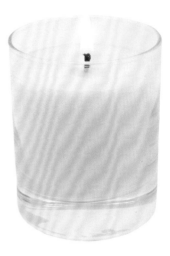

• **Yoga**—especially restorative and gentle styles—can ease anxiety and help you sleep better. Take a class two to three times a week to relieve stress and tension.

• **Mindfulness practices and mental health treatments** like cognitive behavioral therapy (CBT) can be very effective in managing the mood swings, depression, and anxiety that often accompany menopause by helping you train your brain to stay positive, handle stress more effectively, and better regulate your emotions. And therapy can give you a safe place to discuss all the changes that are rocking your world.

Just Remember: You'll Get Through It

True, menopause isn't the most fun you'll ever have with your body. But I swear to you that there is a light at the end of the hormonal tunnel. I, and so many other women before me, have managed—with a little help from modern medicine and a lot of help from our friends—to break on through to the other side.

And that's when the magic begins.

12 Small Steps to Tame TMT

❶ Don't smoke.

❷ Maintain a healthy weight.

❸ Exercise daily, including vigorous workouts a few times a week.

❹ Eat plenty of veggies, fruits, and whole grains, and aim for minimal fat and sugar.

❺ Dress in layers to help combat hot flashes.

❻ Go to bed early so you can get plenty of sleep—even if the night sweats hit.

❼ Keep your bedroom cool and bed-clothes light to minimize night sweats.

❽ Ask for help if you're feeling down.

❾ Find a relaxation practice that works for you, whether it's massage, yoga, deep breathing, meditation—or all of the above. And use it regularly.

❿ Have more sex, not less.

⓫ Address any symptoms as soon as they arise.

⓬ Talk with your doctor!

Demystifying Menopause

Like it or not, menopause will change your world. So consider this a great opportunity to take charge of your life and build healthy habits that will pay off now and for years to come.

INSTEAD OF IGNORING THE SIGNS OF MENOPAUSE,

Get to know them. Accepting that menopause is inevitable—and planning for it—will help ease you into this major life transition.

INSTEAD OF SUFFERING IN SILENCE,

Talk about it. Chat with your doctor, partner, girlfriends, and women online. You are not the first woman to go through this, so don't struggle with problems other women have solved. Ask questions, do research, and reach out. The more you know, the better you'll feel.

INSTEAD OF WAITING FOR THE TRAIN TO HIT,

Get moving. Establishing the fundamental habits of a healthy lifestyle now—a plant-based diet, regular exercise, and plenty of sleep—will give you a solid foundation for weathering hormonal upheavals during menopause. What's more, it will protect your heart, bones, and overall health for the rest of your life.

INSTEAD OF SAYING, "HECK, NO!" TO HORMONE REPLACEMENT THERAPY,

Say, "Maybe." HRT isn't for everyone, and it does have some health risks. However, it has been a big help for many women, especially those who are truly suffering from their symptoms. So don't rule it out without talking to your doc about your particular circumstances.

INSTEAD OF GIVING UP ON SEX BECAUSE IT'S UNCOMFORTABLE,

Lube up and have more sex! For mild vaginal dryness, try over-the-counter lubricants or vaginal moisturizers, which are easy to use and work well. If that's not enough, talk with your gynecologist about local estrogen therapy in the form of a vaginal ring, tablet, or cream, to help relieve dryness and irritation. Unlike HRT, this won't address systemic problems, like hot flashes and mood swings, but it has much lower risks, too. Staying sexually active helps keep your vagina in shape and increases blood flow, which increases lubrication.

INSTEAD OF LETTING MENOPAUSE RULE YOUR LIFE,

Take control! If ever there was a time to eat well, move your body, sleep more, and connect with your best girlfriends, it's right now.

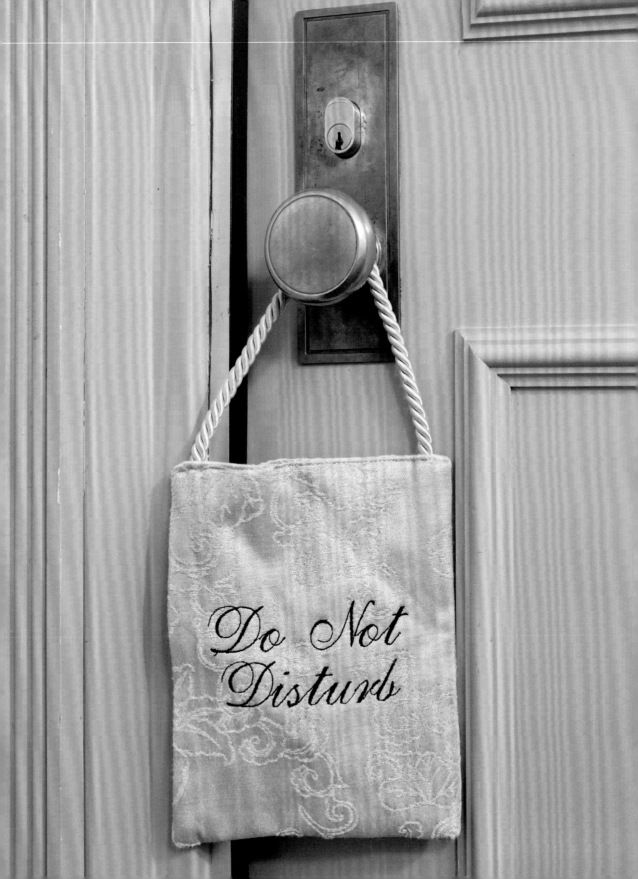

CHAPTER 6

Better Living Through Better Sex

"At 74, I have never had such a fulfilling sex life."

—JANE FONDA

Jane Fonda may sound too cool when she brags about enjoying sex well into her 70s. But why shouldn't she enjoy it? Just because we're getting older, are we supposed to suddenly lose interest? Pretend we no longer have sex? No longer want it?

Absolutely not! The reality is that sex can be even more amazing as we age, because we, dear readers, are at the top of our game. Think about it: You're not worried about getting pregnant, you've had decades to discover what you like, and you aren't (or shouldn't be) afraid to coach your partner. You're finally at that delicious time of your life when you can feel free to actually say—out loud—that, yes, you love sex and want more of it!

Sure you can live well and be happy without sex, and it might just be something you're not interested in. But, if you are, sex is a lovely part of a healthy life. And if like me, you've lived most of your life being a bit more shy about sex than Ms. Fonda, well … get over it! It's time, girlfriends, to reclaim a part of you that can be absolutely fantastic.

Besides, it's good for you.

Want to Look and Feel Amazing?

While most of us enjoy sex because it feels good, it also offers some very nice benefits beyond just making our cheeks glow. And, far from being less important as we get older, regular sex can actually help us age better. If you need a few good reasons to jump in the sack (alone or otherwise), here you go:

• Arousal and orgasm help to increase oxytocin (the feel-good hormone) and decrease cortisol (the stress hormone), leading to better sleep.

• According to researchers in Scotland, people who have sex around three times a week actually look (and feel) younger, due to hormones like estrogen and oxytocin that are released during sex—and they probably take better care of themselves, too. What are you waiting for?

• Sexual arousal and orgasm cause blood to flow to the vaginal walls, making them more lubricated and elastic. You may need a little help from prescription or over-the-counter lubricants to get started, but having sex a few times a week can keep things flowing along nicely.

• Couples who touch each other more frequently—it doesn't have to be intercourse—tend to report higher marital satisfaction than those who do not, even after many years of being together. And if you *are* thinking sex: A 2015 study from the Society for Personality and Social Psychology found that the happiest couples were those who reported having sex at least once a week—although doing it more often didn't make them any happier. (But it didn't make them *less* happy, either ...)

• Studies show the pain of headaches—even migraines—can be lessened by having an orgasm. Our blood pressure drops after sex, which can reduce tension headaches, and the endorphins triggered by orgasm are powerful natural painkillers. In

Nitric Oxide: The Sexy Health Boost?

According to Christiane Northrup, a leading authority on women's health, nitric oxide is one reason sex is so good for us. It is released from the lining of our blood vessels during intercourse and orgasm, which increases blood flow to organs, reducing cellular inflammation. Inflammation can wreak all kinds of havoc in our bodies, and may contribute to cancer, heart disease, arthritis, Alzheimer's, osteoporosis, and autoimmune disease. So three cheers for a good romp in the hay, eh?

> ## *Good sex is like good bridge. If you don't have a good partner, you'd better have a good hand."*
> —MAE WEST

fact, regular sex can almost double our overall pain tolerance, according to recent studies from Rutgers University.

• People who have sex a few times a week are happier than those who rarely do. Those magical endorphins and oxytocin, along with other hormones, not only make them feel good but also make them feel good about themselves.

• The more sex you have, as it turns out, the more you want. It's even more addictive than French fries. (Lower calories, too …) So if it's been a while, then it's time to talk to your partner about how to get things started again. And if you don't have a partner, then book a little "me time" and rediscover just how good it feels to feel good.

• Having intercourse, especially with orgasm, exercises and strengthens the pelvic-floor muscles, which not only increases the pleasure of sex but also can help keep you from becoming incontinent.

• To lower blood pressure, it's not just arousal or orgasm that does the trick, but actual sexual intercourse, which offers a nice burst of aerobic exercise.

• Okay, it's not quite a substitute for a real cardio session, but active sex is still a fun way to burn extra calories. Researchers at the University of Montreal sent young couples home with fitness monitors and discovered that the average woman burns 3.1 calories during every minute of sex. And the friskier your fun, the better the workout.

"Men love women who love sex."

—ESTHER PEREL

Sex Ed Redux: What's Really Happening Down There?

Do you remember the day your teachers separated the boys from the girls and took you to different classrooms for "the talk"? For most of us, that discussion stuck to the basics about where babies come from and how to use a maxi pad. But it probably left out all the juicy details about sex—including how it actually works.

The physiology of sex is pretty straightforward and, like sleep, has well-defined phases:

Excitement, also known as initial arousal or foreplay. In women, this is when the clitoris begins to swell and the vagina begins producing a lubricating liquid; in men, the penis starts to become erect.

Plateau, or full arousal. In both men and women, the heart rate rises, blood flow increases, breathing may become more rapid, and muscles begin to tense.

Orgasm. The climax of all the excitement: The muscles in and around both the vagina and penis contract, creating a variety of extremely pleasurable sensations.

Resolution. Post-orgasm, men and women both experience overall relaxation and a drop in blood pressure as heart rate and breathing slow back down to normal and all those happy hormones come flooding out. In men, the penis will slowly become more flaccid and, during what is called the refractory period, they will be unable to have another orgasm for at least an hour. Most women do not have a refractory period and can have more than one orgasm during any given sexual experience. Lucky us!

Safe Sex at Every Age

Who needs to practice safe sex? Anybody who is having sex. End of story.

Even if you are postmenopausal and no longer concerned with preventing pregnancy, you still need to worry about sexually transmitted diseases (STDs).

Believe it or not, STDs are on the rise again, especially in older populations. Between 2000 and 2015 the rates of gonorrhea, syphilis, and chlamydia infection more than doubled among Americans 45 and over. And, according to the CDC, 26 percent of all new HIV infections diagnosed in 2011 occurred in people over 55.

You're Never Too Old

Even though depictions of sexuality in popular culture focus almost exclusively on the sub-30 crowd, sex can be a lifelong pleasure. And despite physical changes that come with age, clinical studies (and chats with my girlfriends) have established that most women over 45 do not—I repeat, *do not*—have trouble achieving orgasm. It might take longer, but that's not so bad, is it?

Why Are These Numbers Going Up?

• After they go through menopause and no longer have to worry about preventing pregnancy, many women quit asking their partners to use condoms.

• Normal postmenopausal changes, like the drying and thinning of the vaginal walls, make older women even more susceptible to STD infection.

• The introduction of pharmaceuticals like Viagra and Addyi has made it easier to overcome physical obstacles to sex. More sex = more STDs.

• Because we're living longer, many of us are reentering the dating world after losing a partner to death or divorce, and we might not be as sex-savvy—or as safe—as younger generations.

Even more scary? Older people are the least likely to use condoms. A study of sexual health from Indiana University found the lowest rates of condom use were among those 45 and older, and according to research, only 6 percent of sexually active adults age 61 and older use them! While that's fine for couples in long-term monogamous relationships where both partners have been faithful and tested, it is absolutely not fine for everybody else.

So before you start stripping, make sure that both you and your potential sexual partners have been tested for the basics: HIV, HPV, chlamydia, gonorrhea, syphilis, and hepatitis. There is no single good test for herpes, but you'll definitely want to discuss it with your partner if either of you has ever had an outbreak. Make sure you both have either a clean bill of health or a solid plan for preventing transmission of any disease. It might be an awkward conversation, but here's the rule: If a would-be lover won't talk, you walk.

If you're both in the clear and you've been in a monogamous relationship for at least three months (and if your doctor confirms that you're past menopause), then you're probably safe to skip the protection. But if you or your partner has sex with anybody else—even once—you're going to need to start all over.

Where, Oh Where, Did That Libido Go?

If you're in an otherwise happy relationship and used to enjoy sex but now don't care, the odds are good something specific has caused your sex drive to plummet.

First things first: Check in with your doctor. While a low sex drive is a legitimate medical concern on its own, it may also be a red flag for other issues. Several common health problems can squash libido, ranging from a thyroid imbalance to heart disease. Several medications are also known to reduce sex drive, including—ironically—some types of hormonal birth control. Even lower hormone levels due to menopause can reduce your interest in canoodling.

All of these things can be fixed with a little help, so getting them treated can start you on the way to rekindling that spark.

WHAT ABOUT THE LITTLE PINK PILL?

In 2015 the FDA gave approval for a drug called Addyi, which was developed to increase libido in women with low sex drive. However, Addyi has been controversial from the start, because it was only marginally effective and demonstrated a host of serious side effects, like nausea, dizziness, fainting, and low blood pressure. These problems are even worse for women who drink alcohol, use hormonal birth control, or take several common medications. Bottom line? It is an option, but many women and their doctors have concluded that the skimpy benefits aren't worth the risks.

Playtime for Grown-Ups

Although all the phases of sex can be enjoyable, sometimes we need a little extra time and stimulation to get to the big payoff. Regardless of age, an estimated 70 percent of women need direct clitoral stimulation in order to orgasm, so vaginal intercourse alone doesn't always do the trick.

One solution—and a very good one at that: Bring on the toys! Vibrators, dildos, and other sexy playthings can enhance the experience of sex.

On February 17, 2014, Barbara Walters, then 84, shocked not only her TV audience but her fellow cohosts on *The View* when she admitted to owning and using a vibrator she had nicknamed Selfie. While some people—including the usually outspoken Whoopi Goldberg—said Walters's confession was TMI, I felt otherwise. Here was a well-respected older woman speaking publicly about her own sexual pleasure. You go, girl!

But there's nothing new about sex aids. Archaeologists have discovered dildos from as far back as the Stone Age, and the first handheld electric vibrators—excuse me, "personal massagers"—were patented in 1902.

Since then, the devices have become so commonplace that a 2009 study published in the *Journal of Sexual Medicine* found that almost 53 percent of women between 18 and 60 had used a vibrator. And why not? Vibrators can provide the clitoral stimulation that most women need to climax, and women who use them report enhanced sex lives. Need more proof you're not alone? As of 2014, people spent $15 billion a year on sex toys. And that figure is projected to rise to more than $50 billion a year by 2020.

Experimenting with vibrators (or other means) as foreplay can also enhance sex. Many women who bring themselves to orgasm before intercourse report having more intense orgasms during sex with their partners. Try it—it works!

So if you're not enjoying sex as much as you'd like, perhaps your very own personal massager would be a good addition to your nightstand.

Sex by the Numbers

According to a National Center for Health Statistics survey of adults between 25 and 44, women claim an average of four sex partners in their lifetime, while men report an average of seven. (Don't think too hard about that math ...)

Another study found that 19 percent of women and 54 percent of men think about sex every day.

Your Cheating Heart

According to both anthropologist Helen Fisher and sex therapist Esther Perel, people usually don't have affairs because they no longer love their partners. Far more often, men and women have affairs for reasons that are far more complex, often because they've lost something or someone in the previous year or two—like a family member, a house, a job, or some aspect of their identity (like youth).

For both men and women, that sense of loss can be tied up in a big bow and called a midlife crisis. And some of us try to recapture our sense of wholeness—or at least distract ourselves from the loss—by having an affair with someone new.

So if you want to keep your relationship working long-term, do your utmost to fight through the crushes and make that "someone new" the partner you already have.

But What If You Just Aren't in the Mood?

Medical problems aside, for those of us who've been with our partners for more than a few years—or who have an endless to-do list crushing our libido—one of the biggest challenges we face is getting ourselves to want sex. We might love sex once we're having it, but getting there is the problem. So how do we get in the mood?

Spend time apart. Sex expert Esther Perel suggests that couples can boost their mutual attraction to each other if they don't spend all their time together, pursuing (nonsexual!) interests with other people. When you try to be everything to each other, you can easily feel stifled and bored.

Make the right kind of space. Perel also advises partners to create an "erotic space" by designating a place and time you can come together as lovers without the distractions of the outside world. Translation: No TV in the bedroom.

Fantasize. Think about things that have worked in the past to turn you on—memories, fantasies, books, movies—whatever it takes.

Plan a sex date. Wanna know a secret? The best sex, Perel says, is planned sex. You can start thinking about it in the days or hours leading up to it—what you'll wear, do, and say—and you can let your imagination run wild, which can be a huge turn-on.

Skip the panties. It sounds so sophomoric, I know, but there's something about going commando—especially under skirts and dresses—that makes you feel totally sexy. And your partner will love it, too.

Quickie turn-on. If you've tried everything and you're still not feeling that loving feeling, go for the thing that hardly ever fails: masturbate. Yes, really. Lock yourself in the bathroom for a few minutes—with or without your vibrator—and get to it. You'll be ready in no time.

Later-Life Loves

Of course, not all women are in a sexual relationship right now. And many of us like it that way. But others might wish they had a partner in pleasure, whether they're single by choice, divorced, or widowed. Whatever the situation, dating works the same way at any age: You have to meet people first, then see if feelings develop. (Unless you're looking for a one-night stand!)

But ... how?

Here are a few tried-and-true ways to make new friends (with or without benefits):

Do what you love. If you follow your own interests, especially by taking classes or joining clubs, you'll meet people who share your passions, and can get to know them without pressure. Even if you don't meet the love of your life, you might meet one of their best friends. Speaking of which ...

Use your network. You don't have to turn dating into a job search, but networking works! The people we hang out with socially tend to share our interests and values, and are vested in our happiness. What's more, according to a 2012 study conducted at Stanford University, approximately 30 percent of straight couples met through mutual friends, about 25 percent met online, and 10 to 20 percent met at work. So if you want to meet people, spread the word. Let people know you're looking. And if Susie Matchmaker wants to send you on a blind date, say yes!

Move It!

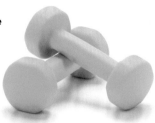

Getting regular exercise of any kind is one of the most reliable ways to improve your sex life and raise your libido. In fact, one study found that exercise was more effective than hormone treatments for increasing sex drive in women—especially if that workout concluded about 30 minutes before sex. Want extra benefits? Exercise with your partner, which has been shown to improve sex for both men and women.

But if you want to enjoy sex even more, adding a few targeted "sexercise" moves to your routine can tone muscles, loosen your hips, and stimulate some sex-craving hormones.

SQUATS help strengthen the thighs, glutes, and lower abdominal muscles and increase mobility in the hips.

BOTH FORWARD AND SIDE-TO-SIDE LUNGES stretch and strengthen the hip and thigh muscles and increase flexibility.

PELVIC LIFTS tone pelvic muscles.

THE BRIDGE POSE further strengthens the thighs, glutes, abdominal, and pelvic muscles—and builds stamina.

PLANKS strengthen arms, thighs, and core muscles to help you support your weight (and your partner!) while engaged in sex.

HAPPY BABY is a simple yoga pose that stretches your hips and lower back. Lie on your back with your feet in the air, bend your knees toward your shoulders, and use your hands to hold onto your legs wherever you can reach—thighs, ankles, or the outside of your feet—pulling your knees down toward the floor while rocking gently from side to side.

KEGEL EXERCISES—contracting, holding, then relaxing the pelvic-floor muscles repeatedly—are often prescribed to help women who are dealing with incontinence. But they can also improve vaginal tone and lubrication, as well as increase the intensity of orgasms. The best part? You can do them secretly anytime, anywhere—including during sex.

Change your routine. If you always get your coffee at the same café, shop at the same grocery store, and lift weights at the same gym, change it up. To meet new people, try going to new places. And when you're there …

Make time for small talk. Getting to know people takes time, and some of the most interesting people don't always catch your eye at first glance. But a pleasant chat might reveal that the helpful bookstore owner or the person sitting next to you on the plane is someone you'd like to know better.

Go digital. Online matchmaking can absolutely work if you aren't meeting promising paramours in your analog life. For best results, stick to the paid sites and consider one aimed at people in your age group or those who share your religion or interests. Ask friends to help you craft your dating profile (they know what's most lovable about you). And give it time. Odds are you will reject and be rejected many times before you meet someone you click with. It's nothing personal. It's just dating.

Have Some Fun

Sex truly is one of life's pleasures, so don't relegate it to the back burner just because you think you think you've "aged out." Take a cue from Jane Fonda (and me!): Grown-up girls really do want to have fun—and at this point, that's really what sex is all about.

10 Small Steps to Sexy Fun

❶ Make a space in your home where you can enjoy sex.

❷ Good sex is planned sex, so get out your calendar.

❸ When your mood needs a boost, just think "sex."

❹ Do Kegels (pelvic-floor exercises) several times a day.

❺ If dryness prevents you from enjoying sex, try an OTC lubricant or talk to your doctor about other prescription options.

❻ Bring out the toys.

❼ Always practice safe sex.

❽ Be bold, brave, and experimental.

❾ If a sexual partner isn't around, learn how to fly solo.

❿ Let sex be what it's meant to be right now: good fun with benefits.

Getting Your Groove On

Sex can be a delicious part of life—for your entire life—if you make it a priority.

INSTEAD OF BEING DISCREET,

Turn yourself into a sexpert. Talk to your partner, talk to your girlfriends, talk to doctors, read books and magazines, and learn everything you can about sex. You don't have to try everything, but at least you'll have options. Feeling retro? Alex Comfort's *The Joy of Sex*—first published in 1972—continues to be a best seller today because it's still chock-full of great ideas.

INSTEAD OF RELEGATING SEX TO THE BEDROOM AND THE END OF THE NIGHT,

Seduce your sweetie in different places and at different times. Try a morning quickie in the kitchen, or an evening plunge in the bathtub. Test out the living room rug, or perch on the bathroom counter. Variety, after all, is the spice of life.

INSTEAD OF STICKING TO THE SAME POSITIONS,

Turn things upside down and sideways. There are many, many ways to have sex, and exploring the many variations together is a bonding experience that will bring you closer to your partner. If you need inspiration, the Kama Sutra is a classic book on sex positions. But just daring each other to try something new once in a while is a serious turn-on for most couples.

INSTEAD OF WAITING FOR A PARTNER,

Please yourself. With or without a vibrator or other toy, masturbation is a great way to enjoy your own body and find out what works for you. *Bonus:* You get all the health benefits of orgasm, too.

INSTEAD OF WAITING FOR THE KIDS TO GO TO BED,

Book a hotel room for date night. Got kids at home (even adult ones)? Escape from parenthood once in a while and run away for a little "we time." Even if it's only for a few hours, there's something crazy-sexy about a secret rendezvous. Got a weekend? Leave the kids with Grandma and Grandpa, and take your romance out of town.

INSTEAD OF CRYING ABOUT AN EMPTY NEST,

Turn your home back into a love nest. If the kids have moved out, give your house a romance makeover. Spruce up your boudoir, upgrade the couch to one that invites spontaneous spooning, and replace the school photos with images that remind you of your playful side, rather than your progeny. You could also take a tip from actress Kyra Sedgwick, who says that after their children left home, she and her husband, actor Kevin Bacon, spiced up their love life by walking around the house naked.

INSTEAD OF THINKING YOU DON'T HAVE TIME FOR SEX,

Schedule some passion. It might seem contrived, but planning a playdate can be the spark that rekindles the habit, especially if you think you're too busy. (*Hot tip:* You aren't.) Put it on the calendar and get to it!

INSTEAD OF TURNING TO STARCHY SNACKS FOR A MOOD BOOST,

Snack on libido lifters and improve your mood the old-fashioned way. Loading up on fruits and vegetables will help you feel strong and energetic enough to get frisky—especially raspberries, watermelon, and fresh figs, which all contain compounds with aphrodisiac properties. You can literally add spice to your life with cloves, ginger, saffron, and ginseng, which all have stimulating effects. And, yes, oysters can boost libido—but so will other zinc-rich foods, like almonds and sesame seeds.

INSTEAD OF FAKING IT,

Ask for what you want. If you aren't having a truly ecstatic experience during sex, gently guide your partner into the positions and moves that drive you wild. And if you don't know what they are, try a little solo experimentation and report back.

INSTEAD OF JUMPING IN COLD,

Set yourself up for romance. If your sex drive needs a little time to warm up, then plan for it—and don't be afraid to go old-school. Light a few candles, put out flowers, and snuggle in next to your sweetie to watch a steamy movie.

INSTEAD OF WORRYING ABOUT HOW YOU LOOK DURING SEX,

Concentrate on your partner and how you are making each other feel. Take turns pleasing each other and give the experience your full attention. An attentive partner is the most attractive partner.

INSTEAD OF MAKING SEX ALL-OR-NOTHING,

Find ways to sneak sexiness into your whole day. Make a point of treating yourself—and your partner—as a sexual person and you'll quickly find that you are having more (and better) sex. Send your partner saucy texts or emails throughout the day. Pick up some massage oil and trade back rubs. Indulge in hugs and kisses every time one of you walks into the house—and don't just peck lips, either. Dress every day in a way that makes you feel like getting undressed, right down to sexy lingerie if you like. And if it's just the two of you at dinner, flirt as if you were on your first date.

INSTEAD OF THINKING ONLY ABOUT YOUR PARTNER'S PLEASURE,

Get selfish! Women often make the mistake of focusing too much on pleasing our partner. Sure, it's a turn-on to see how we turn someone else on, but now's definitely the time to encourage your partner to please you, too.

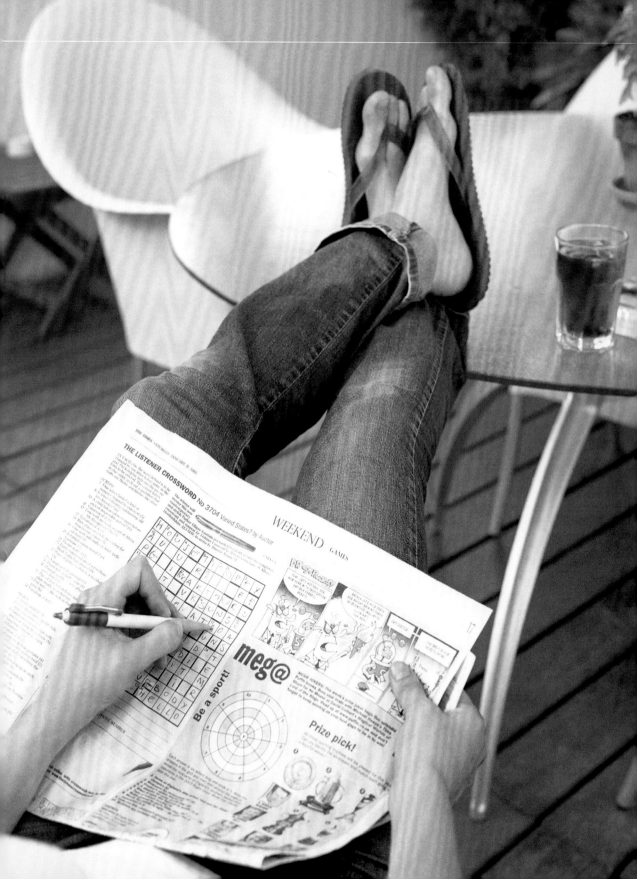

CHAPTER 7

Strong Brain, Sharp Mind

"Biology gives you a brain. Life turns it into a mind."

—JEFFREY EUGENIDES

Confession: My absolute biggest fear is losing my memory. Or my mind. Or both.

Not long ago, I took our dog, Gunther, for one of our frequent walks (good for him *and* for me). Earbuds in, I was chatting with my sister about a movie I'd just seen, while Gunther took care of business. When we got home, I locked the door of my apartment behind me.

I said goodbye to my sister while hanging up my jacket and taking off my walking shoes, then went to the refrigerator for a piece of dark chocolate. (Great for heart and brain health.)

But Gunther was not underfoot, as he normally would be when anyone is in the kitchen. In fact, he was nowhere to be seen. That's when it hit me. I opened the front door, and there he was, waiting patiently for me to finally remember he was still outside. He pranced into the apartment, knowing that a treat would soon be tossed his way.

In my defense, I was distracted by my conversation with my sister. But I didn't feel any less guilty ... or less worried. Was this just normal "brain fog"? Or was it the beginnings of dementia?

The truth is, I was especially concerned because my grandmother died from Alzheimer's at age 81. Toward the end, she no longer recognized her family, and we witnessed her slow, sad decline with grief and fear.

> ## **"Brain power improves by brain use, just as our bodily strength grows with exercise."**
> —A. N. WILSON

Sometimes I forget people's names and, as a writer, there's occasionally a word that gets stranded on the tip of my pen. But that's always been true for me, even when I was in my 20s. And this distinction—whether you're getting more forgetful or have always been that way—turns out to be a crucial bit of information when you're trying to suss out issues with an aging brain.

Gunther forgave me for my brain lapse, and it probably wasn't a sign of anything more serious. But I still want to do everything I can to keep my mind and memory sharp. What's more, I don't just want to protect the brain cells I have; I want to create new ones. (*News flash:* We can!) They say that wisdom comes with age, but I want to get even smarter.

So where the heck did I leave my glasses?

Older Really Does Mean Wiser

Cognitive skills—thinking, memory, learning—change over our lifetime, and new research from Harvard University and MIT shows that some change for the better. Skills like short-term memory, learning, and recalling names peak in our late teens and early 20s. But social understanding (aka people skills) and emotional intelligence continue to improve through our 50s, and vocabulary skills keep getting better around our early 70s.

And here's the really good news: Education, environment, and lifestyle all help preserve your mental skills. The even better news: These are things that are in your control. Take charge of them and you'll help keep your brain in peak condition for life.

What's Going On Up There?

Brains are complicated organs with a huge list of responsibilities. Here are just a few of the things your brain is doing for you right now:

- Regulating your temperature, breathing, and heart rate

- Coordinating your movements and your balance

- Recording, processing, and interpreting sensory information about your environment—and your own body

- Allowing you to think, reason, imagine, dream, and experience emotions

- Cataloging, storing, and retrieving information and memories

- Giving you the ability to speak, read, write, and understand language

These (and many other) functions are spread between the different parts of your brain, which is made up of 100 billion neurons capable of sending and receiving the

What's Normal, Anyway?

Many people incorrectly believe serious mental decline, or senility, is an inevitable part of aging. It's not. Mild memory loss, however—emphasis on mild—*is* normal, so if you can't remember the name of somebody you met just last night, you've got plenty of company. By the time we reach 50, over half of us experience a little forgetfulness (sorry, Gunther), and we all see a deterioration of short-term memory as we get older.

The key is whether your memory lapses are growing significantly more frequent and if you're forgetting the kinds of things you used to remember. For example, have you always had trouble with lists, directions, or where you put things? No need to panic. Suddenly forgetting your address three times a week? That may be a problem.

So if you forget something trivial now and then, just try to relax. (No, really: Relax. Stress actually affects the way our brains process memories.)

electrochemical impulses that enable everything you do. Protecting these neurons and the connections between them—known as synapses—is critical to keeping our brains healthy as we get older.

Your Brain Through the Years

These changes to your brain over time are normal:

- It shrinks a bit, especially in the hippocampus and prefrontal cortex, which both handle memory and learning.

- Connections between neurons may weaken.

- Blood flow may be reduced.

- Small deposits of plaque and other debris may build up.

- Minor damage may accumulate from inflammation, injury (like concussions), and free radicals.

However, there's a lot you can do to reduce the impact of these unavoidable changes and avoid more serious damage. Some of the most important?

Take good care of your heart. Your brain relies on a steady blood supply, so anything that reduces blood flow will impact brain health.

Does Leg Power = Brain Power?

Here's an intriguing link. Two experiments found a correlation between leg strength and cognitive ability. The first, a Japanese study published in 2014, found a simple way to test brain health: Balance on one leg. If you can't stand on one leg for at least 20 seconds, talk to your doctor. It may indicate damage to small blood vessels in the brain and an increased risk for cognitive decline. A separate British study published in 2015 tracked 150 pairs of twins for a decade and found that the twin who had stronger legs at the beginning of the study showed fewer age-related changes in his or her brain down the line.

Don't smoke. Smoking is correlated with damage to memory, learning, and reasoning, and may increase your risk of dementia. It also increases your risk of heart disease and stroke, both of which impact brain health.

Keep your weight in check. Obesity has been correlated with reduced cognitive performance, and brain scans of obese people showed abnormal damage to the insulation that protects neurons.

Stay active—mentally and physically. Regular aerobic exercise keeps your heart healthy, of course, but it also boosts the areas of the brain that handle memory and learning. And keeping your brain working by providing regular mental challenges—like learning French or taking up the trombone—can actually build new brain cells and create new neural connections.

You Must Remember This

It'll come to me. We've all had the experience of having a word we can't quite get out or an answer that stays just out of reach. This is totally normal and has little to do with age. Our response rates do slow as we get older, but most people are still able to remember the information within a minute or so.

Top of mind. The memories we access more often are easier to recall. Also, those that stimulate strong emotions or involve more than one sensory receptor in the brain—taste, smell, touch, sight—are less likely to be forgotten.

The Feminine Advantage

It's not your imagination: When it comes to memory, women definitely have the advantage over men.

In 2015, *JAMA Neurology* published a study of more than 1,000 men and women that showed that, on average, males' memory really is worse than females'—especially after 40—and that the part of men's brains that controls memory is smaller than that part in women.

Why? Women have more of certain hormones, including estrogen, that protect the memory centers of the brain. We also have a lower overall risk for high blood pressure and cardiovascular disease, which affect brain health over time. Lucky us!

In With the New
So You
Don't Get Old

While doctors used to assume we couldn't build new brain cells, current research shows that isn't true. In fact, in the same way that challenging your body with exercise helps you build fresh muscle cells, continuing to push your mind will help you build new brain cells and more synaptic connections. Just keeping active and engaged can slow age-related damage to your brain, but there are specific strategies to boost your intelligence. And all these extra cells and connections don't just make you smarter; they also act as a safety mechanism called a cognitive reserve, which means that if one part of the brain is injured, other parts may be able to take over its job.

In a sense, every new idea or experience is like a workout for your brain. And the best way to get more workouts is simply to try new things. Want some ideas?

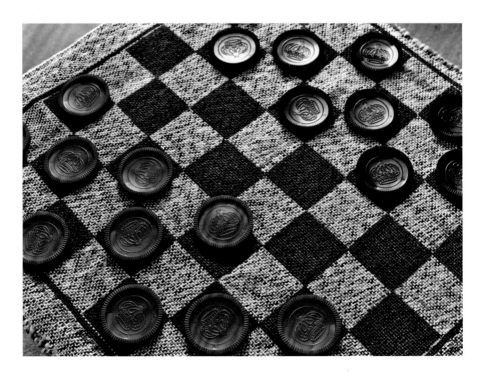

JOIN A CLUB. Interpersonal interaction with a wide array of people is a great way to fire up your brain. Opt for something related to an existing hobby, or get even more mental stimulation by pursuing a brand-new interest.

COOK A NEW RECIPE. Take a class, braise your way through Julia Child's books, or learn to make tamales from a friend. Whatever you do, don't just keep boiling the same spaghetti every Wednesday night.

LEARN A NEW LANGUAGE. Bonus points if it's an immersion class or one that requires a lot of conversation, forcing you to work on your social skills, too. If you travel, make a point to learn at least the basics of the local language. Or consider sign language, which is also good for eye-hand coordination.

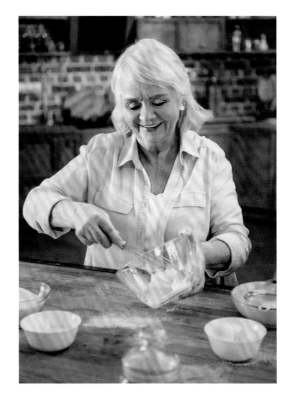

CONFRONT YOUR FEARS. Take a drawing class, even if you flunked fifth-grade art. Attend a slide show on the Himalaya, even if heights make you dizzy. Instead of letting your life shrink as you age, keep expanding it with new activities and hobbies.

TAKE UP A SPORT YOU'VE NEVER TRIED. Sure, golf is fine, but why not consider rock climbing, cross-country skiing, or stand-up paddleboarding? Moving your body in new and unaccustomed ways will force your brain to build a new set of neural connections— especially if it challenges your balance or coordination.

PLAY A GAME. Scrabble, chess, and other strategy-based games that involve both mental skills and social interaction can enhance intelligence.

GET YOUR HEART PUMPING! A Swedish study showed that better cardiovascular fitness is associated with increased verbal intelligence. Running is my fave, but skipping rope will challenge your coordination for an extra workout.

"The measure of intelligence is the ability to change."

—ALBERT EINSTEIN

However, as estrogen levels decline during and after menopause, women often become more forgetful, too.

Bonus: The same study concluded that typical memory decline, which begins for both genders when we're in our 30s and gives us occasional minor memory lapses, like forgetting names (and dogs), is not connected to brain disorders and is probably not evidence of Alzheimer's disease.

The D-Word

While almost all of us will experience a small decline in our ability to process and retrieve memories as we age, some of us may develop a more serious form of memory loss known as dementia. It's a scary topic, but it's important to understand what dementia is and how to reduce your risk.

DEMENTIA

Dementia is not a disease per se but a group of symptoms that affect multiple mental functions, including memory, language, problem-solving, and reasoning.

Dementia is not inevitable, although the likelihood of developing it increases with age. You can inherit a predisposition toward dementia, but genetics do not guarantee that any individual will or will not develop it. Dementia is the result of damage to nerve cells in the brain and is caused by a variety of conditions, the most common being Alzheimer's disease, which may account for 60 to 80 percent of cases. Vascular disease and stroke, Parkinson's disease, Huntington's disease, depression, and chronic drug use are also associated with dementia, which is why dementia may sometimes have more than one cause.

Early signs of dementia are easily overlooked and include episodes of forgetfulness, trouble keeping track of time, and losing one's way in familiar settings. As the condition progresses, these episodes increase in frequency and severity, and a person may find it harder to recognize faces and remember names or words. She may repeat questions, neglect basic hygiene, and appear increasingly sloppy or unkempt. In advanced dementia, people can't care for themselves at all and may be obviously withdrawn, depressed, or even aggressive.

SO WHAT IS ALZHEIMER'S DISEASE?

Alzheimer's is a progressive and fatal disease of the brain, which robs a person of mental and physical function over the span of several years. Scientists don't know exactly what causes it, and there is currently no cure, although there is much ongoing research. What is known is that people with advanced Alzheimer's have fewer brain cells than healthy people, and fewer connections between brain cells. Evidence suggests that protein deposits may accumulate and form plaques and tangles in the brain that interfere with brain cell communication and reduce nutrient delivery. As a result, the affected cells die off.

Symptoms of Alzheimer's develop over time, but neurological damage may begin many years before the first symptoms appear. At present there is no conclusive test for Alzheimer's, but a skilled doctor using memory tests, brain scans, blood samples, and other clinical tools can often diagnose the disease. A small minority of Alzheimer's cases have a genetic component, but there is presently no way to be sure

Alzheimer's by the Numbers

• Alzheimer's is the sixth-leading cause of death in the United States and was responsible for more than 93,000 deaths in 2014 alone.

• Approximately 5.5 million Americans are living with Alzheimer's today. That number is projected to reach 16 million by 2050 as our population ages.

• One in nine Americans 65 and over, and nearly one in three Americans over

age 85, has been diagnosed with Alzheimer's. Early-onset Alzheimer's accounts for less than 10 percent of all cases.

• From the point where symptoms become noticeable, most people with Alzheimer's decline gradually over eight to 10 years.

• Fifteen million adults are responsible for providing or arranging care for a person with Alzheimer's.

True or False?

Memory loss can happen to anyone.

True. Both genetics and chance play a role in dementia and other forms of memory loss. But lifestyle factors like diet, exercise, and stress management can either increase or reduce your risk.

My brain hasn't changed since I was a teenager.

False. The production of proteins involved in forming new memories decreases as we get older. The good news is that regular physical exercise and mental challenges enhance brain function, no matter how old we are.

I'd notice if I had memory loss.

False. Among people diagnosed with mild Alzheimer's, 42 percent didn't know anything was wrong.

Diet affects brain health.

True. People who eat lots of fruits and vegetables, fish, nuts, and olive oil may be less likely to develop thinking and memory problems. Regardless, it's *always* a good idea to keep a healthy diet.

A healthy body holds a healthy mind.

True. Being overweight in middle age has been tied to a higher risk of dementia. High cholesterol may also be associated with mild memory loss and cognitive decline. Treating these conditions can help lower that risk.

Women are more likely to develop Alzheimer's than men.

True. Women are twice as likely as men to get Alzheimer's. It has been suggested, but not confirmed, that the hot flashes that come with menopause increase cortisol production, which can impair memory. Another reason: Alzheimer's risk increases with age, and women tend to live longer than men.

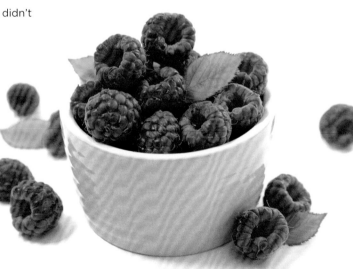

whether or not a particular person will develop the disease even if he or she has the genetic markers.

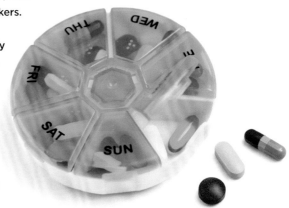

More than five million Americans are currently living with Alzheimer's, and the disease is on the rise, largely because we are living longer. Since there is no cure, it is treated with support services to help people maintain the best possible quality of life.

What's New in Alzheimer's Research?

More than 100 years after Alzheimer's was officially described, experts continue to be confounded about why it happens and how to stop it. But Harvard researchers recently unveiled a very promising theory about what causes plaque in the brain—which seems to always be present in people with Alzheimer's. It seems that infections—viral, bacterial, or fungal—in the body (even those that are mild enough to be undetected) can create a strong reaction that leaves debris in the brain, which then causes plaque to build. This discovery could be the game-changer researchers have been looking for, helping to find ways to prevent and even cure this dreadful disease.

In another big breakthrough, researchers at UCLA have developed a therapeutic program—not a drug—that may be able to reverse some of the memory loss associated with Alzheimer's, particularly for those in the early stages. The therapy relies on a comprehensive series of healthy lifestyle changes that includes eliminating processed foods, eating more fish, meditating, practicing yoga, doing brain-stimulating exercises, and getting plenty of sleep and physical exercise. The first small clinical trial ended in 2014 with nine out of the 10 participants showing noticeable improvements, which they continued to sustain after the trial ended. Larger studies are under way now, but additional evidence from UCLA research suggests that healthy habits like those outlined in this book may help reduce the risk of Alzheimer's.

Not All Memory Loss Is Dementia

Alzheimer's and dementia are frightening, but there are more than 50 common disorders that can cause dementia-like symptoms in people over 45. In these cases, the symptoms usually disappear when the underlying condition is treated. Watch out for memory loss and mental confusion related to:

Drugs and drug interactions. Many common medications can cause temporary memory loss. What's more, if you take multiple medications, including prescription and over-the-counter drugs or supplements, they may interact with each other to cause side effects that resemble the symptoms of Alzheimer's and other forms of dementia. Read the warning labels on any medication you take and if you spot any change in your health, alert your pharmacist or doctor and ask them to find alternatives or adjust dosages to mitigate side effects.

Thyroid disease. Unusually high or low levels of thyroid hormone, caused by an over- or underactive thyroid gland, can trigger symptoms that can be mistaken for dementia, such as anxiety or depression, irritability, and forgetfulness or confusion. Low thyroid levels are quite common in postmenopausal women and can be easily treated with medication. An overactive thyroid is less common and may require surgery but is usually also treatable. Either condition can be diagnosed with a simple blood test, so include it with your regular health checks.

Vitamin deficiency. A lack of vitamin B_{12} may result in memory problems and difficulty thinking. Since B_{12} is primarily found in animal products, some vegetarians and vegans might not get enough while people with certain autoimmune conditions might not absorb it effectively through their digestive tract. However, the condition is usually easy to treat by taking B_{12} supplements, either orally or by injection.

Type 2 diabetes. In addition to other complications, diabetes can damage blood vessels in the brain, which can result in memory loss and confusion. A healthy diet, regular exercise, and weight management can often prevent diabetes in the first place. However, if it is already present, it can be managed with diet and medications, which may also relieve memory problems.

Depression. Depression can affect your memory, thinking, mood, and sleep, leaving you feeling mentally dull, foggy, and forgetful. Depression can usually be treated successfully with the help of a doctor. *(See Chapter 12.)*

These and many other problems—including lack of sleep and excessive stress—can mimic the signs of mental decline, so it's important to pay close attention to your overall health and call in an expert if anything doesn't seem right.

When Should I Worry?

As a rule of thumb, if you're worried about your memory, you probably don't have a problem. However, if your friends and family are worried, then it may be serious.

It's time to see a doctor if you find that your typical behavior has begun to change and you are frequently:

- Getting lost in familiar places

- Having difficulty handling money

- Mixing up people, places, or names

- Misplacing objects, particularly in odd places, like putting keys in the freezer

- Leaving tasks or chores undone

- Getting distracted easily

- Losing your place or asking, "Where was I?" when you're reading or talking

Don't panic about small episodes of absentmindedness—especially if they're normal for you, but do get checked out if you recognize yourself having more severe

Proceed With Caution

A study published in *JAMA* found evidence that several OTC antihistamines, pain relievers, and sleep aids, as well as certain prescription drugs used to treat anxiety, depression, and bladder control, are linked to dementia and cognitive impairment. Short-term use does not appear to cause a problem, but higher dosages and more than three years of use raise the risk of long-term damage.

Be especially careful if you're taking any medication with the following ingredients: amitriptyline, atropine, chlorpheniramine, desipramine, dicyclomine, diphenhydramine, hydroxyzine, hyoscyamine, imipramine, meclizine, nortriptyline, olanzapine, oxybutynin, paroxetine, prochlorperazine, promethazine, pseudoephedrine hydrochloride/triprolidine hydrochloride, scopolamine, or tolterodine.

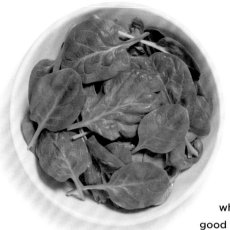

or frequent lapses. Odds are good that it's a symptom of something easily treatable, but if it is more serious, the sooner you get evaluated, the better your long-term prognosis will be.

Chew on This

Your brain uses 20 percent of your body's energy supply, so it's important to keep it well nourished. But what to eat? Well, whatever's good for your heart is also good for your brain.

A recent study from the Mayo Clinic found that simply eating fewer than 2,150 calories a day was linked to better brain health. Diets emphasizing fresh veggies, whole grains, beans, nuts, and fish (and a daily glass of red wine!) have been shown to contribute to brain health. In one study, researchers at Columbia University found that people who ate a veggie-heavy Mediterranean diet had more brain volume than people eating a more typical American diet, with lots of processed foods, saturated fat, and starchy carbs.

As you plan your meals, be sure to include plenty of these proven brain boosters:

Folate. Low levels of this B vitamin are linked to a higher risk of stroke, which can sometimes be a cause of dementia. *Find it in:* Beans, spinach, and fortified whole grains.

Staying Sharp:
Your Guide to a Brain-Smart Life

Here's a bright idea. AARP offers a terrific online tool to help you stay on top of your mental game. The program, Staying Sharp, uses a science-based approach that starts with a personalized assessment to measure key aspects of your brain health. It then gives you specific tips to help you change your behavior, all based on five key strategies: move, discover, relax, nourish, and connect. Check it out at *www.stayingsharp.org* and remember—the sooner you start, the sharper you'll stay.

Vitamin E. Many people suffering from memory loss have been found to be deficient in this essential nutrient, suggesting that vitamin E's antioxidant properties may protect brain cells against damage from the destructive molecules known as free radicals. *Find it in:* Seeds, nuts, oils, and tomatoes.

Vitamin K. In older adults, higher levels of vitamin K are associated with improved episodic memory—like remembering where you left your keys. *Find it in:* Herbs, leafy or stalky vegetables like broccoli and kale, salad greens, asparagus, leeks, and soybeans.

Don't Fear the F-Word

The F-word in this case is "forgetfulness." Ordinary memory loss affects most of us, but these simple strategies can help you minimize the effects on your day-to-day life:

• To keep track of important information and dates, keep a calendar and a to-do list in either a paper or digital notebook. And use them!

• Designate a place for your keys, phone, glasses, and purse or wallet, and put them in the same place each and every day. You're less likely to forget where things are if they are always in the same spot!

• Get enough quality sleep—that's seven to nine hours a night. Lack of sleep contributes to a host of memory problems.

• Cut back on alcohol.

• Cultivate a good sense of humor. Stressing makes memory loss worse!

• Build yourself a palace: An ancient but effective technique for remembering lists or items is to create a "memory palace" in your mind by associating the things you want to remember with the various rooms. The trick is to create a series of imaginary scenes so vivid and outrageous that you can't forget them—and to lock in the memories with sensory details. For instance, you might recall a grocery list by picturing yourself opening your front door, which is painted with gooey peanut butter, then walking across a doormat made of grainy whole wheat bread, and continuing into the hallway, where you stumble over a pile of sweet potatoes. When you are ready to recall the list, just re-create your mental movie and get shopping!

Omega-3 fatty acids. These essential oils improve memory and brain function. *Find them in:* Seafood like salmon, shrimp, halibut, mackerel, sardines, trout, and fresh tuna (your mother was right—fish are brain food!); nuts and seeds; and supplements or specially enriched foods.

Blueberries. Blueberries are rich in antioxidants, which support heart health but also appear to increase communication between neurons and may even help with balance and coordination.

Dark chocolate. Dark chocolate with at least 70 percent cacao has been shown to increase blood flow to the brain and encourage the growth of new brain cells. Is this stuff great or what?

Good Health, Good Smarts

It turns out there's a lot we can do to keep our brains working at full capacity. And one simple rule stands out: What's good for your heart is good for your bones, good for your weight, good for your mood, good for you libido, good for your overall health ... and good for your brain.

---

10 Small Steps to a Brilliant Brain

❶ Keep working or volunteering. Stay engaged with the world.

❷ See friends and family often.

❸ Read as much as possible, including books that challenge your vocabulary or your way of thinking.

❹ Try new activities, especially those that require learning new physical or mental skills.

❺ Eat brain-healthy foods, including vegetables, nuts, fish, and olive oil.

❻ Keep your calorie count low and your weight at a healthy level.

❼ Be careful about which medications you take—and reduce or eliminate your use of sleeping pills.

❽ Establish sleep habits that keep you well rested.

❾ Reduce stress through mindfulness exercises, organizational habits, and a commitment to positive thinking.

❿ Move your body every day.

A Sharper Brain

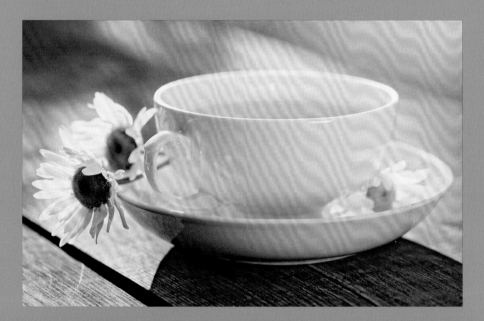

The little choices really do add up. But some of the smartest choices for protecting your brain aren't necessarily obvious.

INSTEAD OF A BACON DOUBLE CHEESEBURGER WITH MAYO,

Choose a black bean burger with guacamole. Opting for plant-based foods and fish instead of meat helps to reduce the risk of heart disease, which also reduces the risk of cognitive decline. And avocados help keep your cardiovascular system healthy and reduce inflammation—both important for brain health.

INSTEAD OF EASING OFF THE WEIGHTS AS YOU AGE,

Bump up your strength training. A recent study found that women who worked out with weights twice a week had less brain shrinkage than those who trained only once a week or did only stretching exercises. And if you aren't regularly working out, get into the habit now. One study says that middle-aged adults who stay in good shape can cut their dementia risk by 40 percent compared to those with low fitness.

INSTEAD OF GOING SOLO ALL THE TIME,

Make a date. People who spend more time with friends have up to 55 percent lower risk of memory problems. On the flip side, loneliness in older people accelerates cognitive decline. Extra credit if your friends are smarter than you—it's one of the best ways to stay sharp and keep learning.

INSTEAD OF RELYING ON THE SAME OLD, SAME OLD,

Surprise yourself. Whether it's taking a different route to work, ordering a different lunch at your local café, or reading a different newspaper, make a point of jumping out of your ruts once in a while. You'll force your brain to work harder and build more neural pathways—and you might find some new favorites, too!

INSTEAD OF PRETENDING YOU KNOW WHAT A WORD MEANS,

Look it up. Increasing your vocabulary also increases your understanding of language, which helps with intellectual tasks and everyday life. What's more, people who exercise their minds by reading, writing, or doing word puzzles have brains that can look younger in scans!

INSTEAD OF JUST LISTENING TO MUSIC,

Learn to play an instrument or take a dance class. Not only will the learning process create new neural pathways in your brain, but music is also a proven mood booster and stress releaser.

INSTEAD OF BUYING YOUR NEXT BLANKET, SCARF, OR HAT,

Make it yourself. Researchers at the Mayo Clinic found that people who picked up handcrafts, like knitting and crocheting, have a decreased risk of developing mild cognitive impairment and memory loss.

INSTEAD OF GOING TO AN ART MUSEUM,

Pick up a paintbrush. A recent German study showed that older people who participate in drawing and painting classes gain increased psychological resilience as well as greater connectivity in areas of the brain associated with cognitive processes like memory. What's more, a Mayo Clinic study found older adults who create original art, like painting or sculpting, are 73 percent less likely to develop mild memory loss.

INSTEAD OF ASSUMING THAT BRAIN DRAIN IS INEVITABLE,

Think positive. In one experiment with younger people, low-achieving students who were encouraged to think that their intelligence could be improved scored better than their peers on tests of the same material.

INSTEAD OF BEING A TECHNOPHOBE,

Use your devices to the max. Set calendar reminders to alert you for birthdays, doctor's appointments, and when to pick up your dry cleaning. Use the alarm on your phone to let you know when to feed the parking meter, and—speaking of parking—use the camera function to take a quick photo of your spot at the mall. The note function on your phone is a great place to keep a running shopping or to-do list.

INSTEAD OF CLUTTERING YOUR COUNTER WITH MEDICINE AND VITAMIN BOTTLES,

Pick up a pillbox organized by days of the week. This will prevent you from skipping medication or doubling up on doses. If you take pills at multiple times of the day, use different pillboxes for morning and night—and label them clearly.

INSTEAD OF GETTING WORKED UP ALL THE TIME,

Chill. Stress releases the hormone cortisol, which can kill brain cells and contribute to premature aging of the brain. And brooding over unpleasant events prolongs these harmful effects.

INSTEAD OF WATCHING CAT VIDEOS ON YOUTUBE,

Stream an online course or TED talk to feed your mind. The Internet is full of great resources—if you use them.

INSTEAD OF VEGGING OUT AFTER DINNER,

Train your brain. In a U.K. study of about 7,000 people, participants age 50 and over showed a significant improvement in reasoning and verbal learning after six weeks of brain-training games and other reasoning tests three times a week. But ordinary puzzles and even complicated knitting or woodworking patterns also help increase focus.

INSTEAD OF WATCHING THE TUBE ALL NIGHT,

Go to bed on time. Poor sleep is linked to mild cognitive impairment, like memory problems. Not to mention that both late nights and excess screen time have been linked to poor sleep.

INSTEAD OF TAKING A SLEEP AID,

Drink herbal tea or warm milk an hour before bed. Both prescription and over-the-counter sleeping pills can cause memory loss, but the naturally occurring tryptophan in milk is a side-effect-free sleep inducer. If dairy doesn't agree with you anymore, brew a relaxing cup of chamomile or catnip tea.

INSTEAD OF POURING ANOTHER DRINK,

Stick to one glass of wine. Some studies have linked moderate alcohol consumption (one drink a day for women and two for men) to a reduced risk of dementia, and resveratrol, found in red wine, has proven antiaging properties. But excess drinking can disrupt your sleep and affect your memory, so moderation matters.

INSTEAD OF ASKING PEOPLE TO SPEAK UP OR SQUINTING AT THE NEWSPAPER,

Get your hearing and vision checked every three years. And use glasses or hearing aids if they're prescribed. If you can't hear or see something, you're surely not going to remember it—and once sensory input becomes limited, cognitive skills may also decline. Besides, the harder your brain has to work to see or hear, the less energy it has for other functions.

INSTEAD OF RETIRING,

Keep working! According to a German study, your career may be keeping your brain healthy. Turns out that a demanding job is to a strong brain what lifting weights is to a strong body. If you don't love your job, find a new one or seek challenging volunteer work instead.

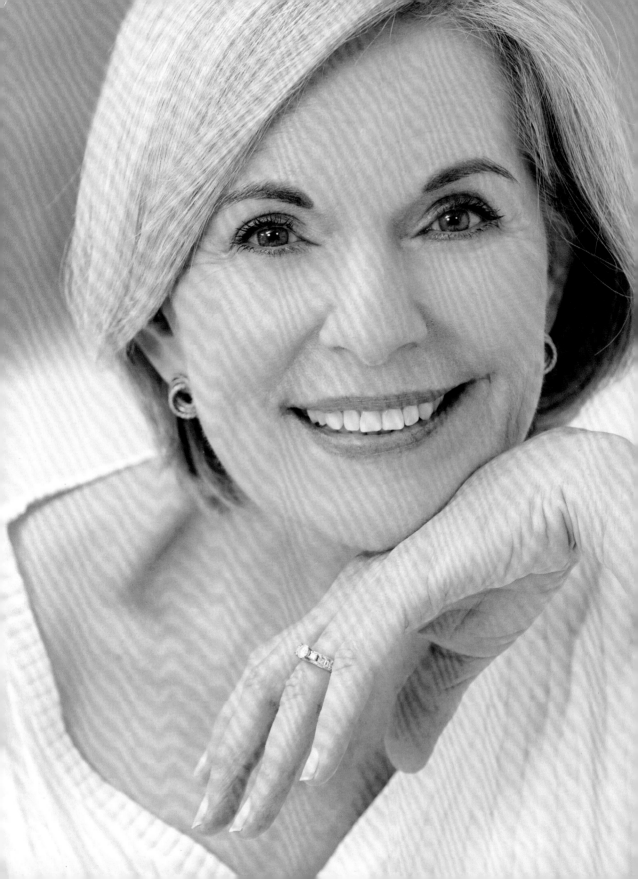

CHAPTER 8

Healthy, Sexy Smile

"[She] laughs at everything you say. Why? Because she has fine teeth."
—BENJAMIN FRANKLIN

It's said that it takes seven seconds to make a first impression. And one of the biggest parts of that impression is your smile. Fair or not, if your teeth aren't aging well, they'll definitely make you look older than you really are.

That's no smiling matter.

Having a beautiful smile—including white teeth and fresh breath—is one of the best ways to seem confident. And no question about it: You'll smile a whole lot more if your grin is as dazzling as you are!

A Healthy Mouth Means a Healthy Body

It's true! Dental care isn't just about looking good; it's also about being healthy. What's going on inside your mouth can affect what's going on inside your body—and it isn't always pretty. In the United States alone, periodontal disease—usually caused by bacteria in the mouth, which results in plaque on teeth—affects one in every two adults, and is the #1 reason people lose their teeth. It can also increase your risk for heart disease, diabetes, and other serious health issues.

Research shows that advanced periodontal disease increases the amount of bacteria in the mouth. The bacteria can then enter the bloodstream and gain access to other parts of the body, causing chronic inflammation and infection. A study conducted in Britain and described in a 2013 issue of the *Journal of Alzheimer's Disease* even found that such bacteria can travel to the brain, potentially causing the kind of brain tissue deterioration that is often seen in patients with Alzheimer's disease.

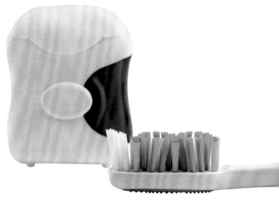

The importance of oral health has been more widely recognized in recent years. In 2000 the Office of the U.S. Surgeon General issued its first-ever oral health report, declaring that "the mouth is the center of vital tissues and functions that are critical to total health and well-being across the life span."

So I think we can agree that keeping the inside of your mouth healthy should be as high a priority as keeping the rest of your body fit. Fortunately, it's not so hard to do.

The Bad News

Regardless of how diligent we are about brushing, almost all of us are going to see signs of aging in our teeth after decades of enjoying a full life. Here's what to expect:

- Teeth get yellow, gray, stained, and worn-down over time. Delicious foods like coffee, tea, red wine, tomato sauces, berries, and beets contribute to the erosion of enamel and the gradual discoloration of our once pearly whites.

- Cavity-prone teeth can feel (and look) like they're filled with metal—and older fillings may be starting to crack.

- Teeth can shift around in your mouth as you age, even if you—like me—wore braces as a kid and diligently followed up those braces with years of wearing a retainer.

- With time and less-than-perfect dental hygiene, our gums can recede when the tissue at the base of our teeth wears away from gum disease, exposing the root of the tooth. (You know that expression "She's a little long in the tooth"?) On the other end, teeth can become worn down from grinding, and chewing on things we shouldn't, like ice.

- Thinning or cracked enamel means teeth become sensitive to everything from that healthy mug of hot green tea to the little scoop of icy-cold gelato you so deserve. Not fun!

The Good News

There are solutions for all of the above!

Simple Habits for a Super Smile

Taking care of your mouth isn't just about looking gorgeous. You need your teeth and mouth to eat, drink, laugh, kiss, speak, sing, whistle, sigh, smile, and do other activities that are essential to your health and happiness. Don't you think they deserve a bit of TLC?

• Visit your dentist every six months for a cleaning and checkup. You probably don't need x-rays every year unless your dentist sees some problems brewing.

• Brush twice a day.

• Floss daily. New evidence indicates that flossing may not be as important as brushing, but it still helps keep your mouth cleaner, smelling fresher, and looking a lot better, too. And it only adds a minute to your routine.

True or False?

Chewing sugarless gum can help prevent tooth decay.

True. While not a substitute for brushing your teeth, chewing on a little sugarless gum helps remove plaque from teeth and increases the flow of saliva.

High-carb foods contribute to tooth decay.

True. Sugary and starchy foods turn to simple sugars in the body, causing cavities and tooth decay. Even some fruit is guilty. Eat a diet full of dark leafy greens and plenty of vegetables to maintain strong teeth.

It's easier to get cavities the older we get.

True. Gums recede with age, exposing the roots of our teeth, which decay faster than the enameled surfaces. In addition to brushing, flossing, and seeing the dentist regularly, drinking lots of water helps to reduce decay-causing bacteria.

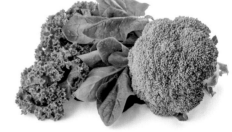

"There was never yet philosopher / That could endure the toothache patiently."
—WILLIAM SHAKESPEARE

• Be vigilant about noticing any changes in your mouth or teeth that might warrant medical attention.

• Have any recommended dental work done pronto. You use your teeth all day, every day, so small problems can get big fast.

Keep It Clean: A Primer

Pardon me for saying so, but your mouth is a hotbed of bacteria. Luckily, that germ factory can be controlled with good oral hygiene.

Floss first. Floss at least once a day *before* brushing your teeth, and anytime you have food stuck between your teeth. For proper form, take an 18-inch strand and, starting at one end, hold a short section between your fingers to floss, moving to a fresh section of the strand after each few teeth. Wrap the floss around each tooth, sliding it as close to the gum line as is comfortable. If you find floss hard to handle, use another interdental cleaner—a flosser, special pick, stick, water cleaner, or brush—to clean between your teeth.

Brush at least twice a day for at least two minutes at a time. At minimum, brush first thing in the

Stop Being So Sensitive!

Sensitivity in our teeth or gums can signify a problem that needs further investigation. Cold sensitivity usually isn't a sign of anything serious and can often reverse itself, so if you feel pain or discomfort when drinking something cold, try switching to a toothpaste for sensitive teeth. But pain triggered by heat could mean a tooth is dying, and, unfortunately, a root canal might be in your future.

morning and before you go to bed. Many electric toothbrushes now have a built-in two-minute timer, but if not, keep an eye on the clock and don't skimp! After meals, wait 30 minutes before brushing—especially if you have acid reflux or you've had something acidic to eat or drink. Acids weaken tooth enamel, and brushing too soon can remove it.

Electric or Manual?

Many dentists recommend electric toothbrushes to help people improve technique and duration of brushing, but according to the Mayo Clinic, there's no significant difference in results as long as you brush thoroughly and consistently.

Harder isn't better. Think of your tooth enamel as fine china and treat it gently. Whether you're using a manual or electric toothbrush, choose one with soft or ultrasoft bristles. Hold the brush at a 45-degree angle, pointed toward the gum line, and methodically brush each tooth: front, back, and chewing surface.

Don't forget your tongue! Scraping your tongue in the morning—before you brush your teeth—removes a significant amount of the bacteria that cause bad breath and other health problems. You could use the edge of a teaspoon, but specially made metal or plastic tongue scrapers are inexpensive, long-lasting, and available at most drugstores. Place the scraper horizontally against the back of your tongue and scrape forward. Rinse the scraper and repeat until your tongue is clean.

Give Yourself a Younger Smile

Is your grin getting dim? It's not just you. It's almost impossible to keep teeth from getting stained over time. But whitening your teeth will take years off your face. And if you do it, you won't be alone. According to the American Academy of Cosmetic Dentistry, whitening is the most requested elective dental procedure. There are lots of ways—from expensive to inexpensive, and from easy to slightly complicated—to get back your 100-watt smile. Here's the skinny:

- All teeth whiteners use some kind of peroxide bleaching solution, with the exception of whitening toothpaste.

• If you have crowns, veneers, or other dental work, they will not be affected by bleach the same way as your regular teeth, so you might end up with mismatched tones.

• All bleaching can increase tooth sensitivity. Although it is usually temporary, it can be painful, especially if you have receding gums. A toothpaste for sensitive teeth can help.

• For the health and the safety of your teeth, be sure to stick to products that are FDA-approved and use them only as directed.

• To avoid damaging teeth and gums, don't bleach more than once a year or according to your dentist's advice.

• Not all stains can be removed. In particular, mineral stains, like those from iron and fluoride, are more stubborn than food, coffee, or wine stains. Some medications can also stain teeth.

• If you have especially stained or pitted teeth, whitening might not be effective; you might want to consider veneers instead.

What About Whitening Rinses and Toothpastes?

We've all seen those ad campaigns promising we can simply brush—or rinse—years of stains away from our teeth. But according to a 2010 study published in the *Journal of Clinical Dentistry,* many whitening toothpastes and oral rinses are very abrasive and can actually strip enamel. And the alcohol in oral rinses can dry out and irritate your mouth and gums. Bottom line: Stick with regular toothpaste and find another way to whiten. You'll save money, and your teeth, too.

TO WHITEN TEETH AT HOME:

Get a tray. The best results you can get at home are by using custom bleaching trays from your dentist. The trays are made specifically to fit your mouth, then you squirt a bleaching gel inside and keep the trays on your teeth for about 30 minutes every day for at least 10 days. Over-the-counter kits with one-size-fits-all trays and a weaker bleaching solution are much less expensive, although they might take longer to produce results.

Pros: Extremely effective against most stains, long-lasting, and considered safe. *Cons:* The cost can be a few hundred dollars for the professional ones from your dentist, but much less for the OTC versions.

OR ...

Do a strip. Many companies sell whitening strips that are placed over teeth for a specified amount of time every day for up to two weeks.

Pros: Easy to use, much less expensive than the trays, and they work pretty well. *Cons:* Not as effective as the whitener you can get from your dentist and requires more frequent touch-up. Also, they might not bleach all the teeth evenly, even compared to OTC trays.

To whiten teeth professionally, get recommendations. Do you admire the beautiful smile of the woman in Accounting at your firm? Ask her how she got it and who did it—or ask your regular dentist for names. Most cosmetic dentists do great work, but the stronger peroxide solution and higher price

What a Grind

Do you ...
- Clench your teeth during the day?
- Grind your teeth at night?
- Have unexplained chips in your teeth or unusually flat front teeth?
- Notice that your front teeth are shorter than they used to be?
- See other unexplained wear and tear on your teeth?
- Have frequent headaches or jaw pain?

If the answer to any of these questions is yes, you might have bruxism (aka tooth grinding), a common problem that often occurs while we sleep. Bruxism can be caused by misaligned teeth, disorders like Huntington's or Parkinson's disease, acid reflux, or other medical conditions, but by far the most common cause is plain old stress.

Left untreated, bruxism can quickly wear down your teeth, destroying enamel, and chipping and cracking teeth, crowns, and even veneers. Not only does it look bad, it opens you up to dental disease as well as painful conditions like temporomandibular joint (TMJ) disorders.

My own dentist diagnosed me with bruxism after he noticed unusual amounts of wear on some of my teeth. So now I am the proud owner of a custom-made mouth guard, which I wear every night to keep my pearly whites from fighting each other. If you notice any of the above symptoms or suspect you're guilty of grinding, check in with your dentist. And maybe we should all try a little more meditation, too.

tag that come with professional bleaching demand that you do your home-work. And don't trust anyone who tries to sell you a blinding-white smile. Artificially bright teeth should stay in Hollywood. A reputable pro will match your teeth to your skin tone for a naturally bright look.

What Else Can You Do?

Almost all of the health risks that threaten our teeth as we age—including prob-lems like receding gums, cavities, infections, and injuries—are going to require professional treatment. So in addition to being diligent about your own dental hygiene, the most important thing you can do for your oral health is to find a qualified dentist you can trust.

But what about the things that just make us look and feel our best? Same answer: A good dentist can give you a whole new reason to smile.

Cracked amalgam fillings? Chances are, if you had a cavity in your early years, it was fixed with a silver amalgam filling. If your amalgam fillings are starting to crack, have them replaced with more modern—and less obvious—porcelain composite fillings that match your teeth. It is possible to have them replaced purely for cosmetic reasons, but most dentists advise wait-ing until a replacement is clinically necessary.

Tooth turning gray? Teeth that have had root canals can sometimes turn gray from the inside out. The whitening formulas that work on external stains won't help, but an endodontist can drill out the filling and apply an internal bleach, which is simple and effective, although it might have to be repeated after a few years.

Crooked or misaligned teeth? If you're suffering from memories of metal grillwork braces, you'll be happy to know that orthodontia has made big strides in recent years. To straighten and realign teeth, you can now use clear aligners that are nearly invisible and are worn all day and night, except when eating. They cost between $3,000 and $8,000 for a full treat-ment and usually take at least a year to work, and you must visit the ortho-dontist for a new set every two or three weeks, but the results are amazing.

Chipped or broken teeth? Nearly any kind of damage can be repaired using porcelain composite that matches your original tooth, whether a

Read My Lips!

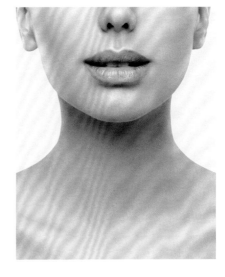

Lips are the gorgeous gateway to your mouth. Keep them soft, kissable, and ready for action.

INSTEAD OF ALWAYS BREATHING THROUGH YOUR MOUTH,
Let your nose do the work. Breathing through your mouth leads to dry mouth, bad breath, and chapped lips.

INSTEAD OF USING YOUR TONGUE TO MOISTEN DRY LIPS,
Stop licking. When you lick your lips, you're smearing them with saliva, which contains enzymes designed to break up food. Here, saliva simply continues trying to do its job by breaking down the surface cells, further aggravating your lips. (And no lip biting, either!) If your pout is feeling parched, either sip water or reach for a moisturizing balm.

INSTEAD OF SUFFERING WITH B-GRADE LIPS,
Bump up your vitamin B. Severely chapped or cracked lips could indicate a vitamin B deficiency. Make sure to include sources like dark leafy greens and almonds in your diet every day and consider a B-complex supplement if you're vegan or vegetarian.

INSTEAD OF LEAVING YOUR LIPS DEFENSELESS,
Slather on the balm. Lip balms act as a protective barrier against cold and wind, and keep moisture from evaporating, so use them several times a day. Look for emollient formulas that include ingredients like beeswax, shea butter, cocoa butter, or food-grade oils such as almond or coconut. And choose lip treatments with an SPF of 30 for maximum protection. Lips can be extremely sensitive to UV rays.

INSTEAD OF LETTING CHAPPED LIPS GET WORSE,
Exfoliate and moisturize. Just as you exfoliate your face and body, you should be doing the same thing for your lips. Scrub them lightly with a soft toothbrush or washcloth—or mix a little plain sugar with a few drops of olive oil, and rub with your fingertips. Rinse, pat dry, then apply balm. Do this every time you exfoliate your face.

small patch or a full crown. The price will vary widely from a couple hundred dollars to fill a chip to well over a thousand dollars for a porcelain crown.

Missing teeth? Whether you've had to have teeth removed or some teeth just never came in, the gap left behind isn't just a cosmetic issue; neighboring teeth tend to lean and shift, and the jawbone deteriorates. Removable dentures or permanent crowns can serve to hold the other teeth in place. But for a solution that also stabilizes the bone, consider implants, in which a steel or titanium post is surgically implanted in your jaw and a porcelain replacement tooth is constructed around the post.

Discolored, pitted, cracked, worn-down, or generally unlovely teeth? Get veneers or get bonded! For veneers, a cosmetic dentist will grind down the front of each tooth, then apply a customized porcelain facade, creating a very natural look that is almost as strong as the original tooth. Bonding is similar but uses a slightly softer resin to create a new surface. Either treatment can change the color, shape, and surface of your teeth. Bonding is among the least expensive options in cosmetic dentistry, starting at around $200 per tooth, but can chip and stain more easily than the alternative. Veneers can cost more than $1,000 per tooth but are long-lasting and very effective in refreshing your look.

Need Another Reason to Make Out?

Kissing is good for your teeth! It's true. Saliva flow increases when we kiss. Saliva also helps to break down oral plaque. Plus the minerals in saliva help build tooth enamel. Each smooch is like a little burst of dental health. Romantic, huh?

A Breath of Fresh Air

Bad breath or halitosis—a faux pas to avoid—can result from such simple causes as improper brushing, lack of flossing, an unclean tongue, or low saliva flow. Saliva is especially important for cleaning your mouth, so reduced saliva flow—usually caused by eating too little—can cause temporary bad breath. However, breath that's persistently less than lovely could be a symptom of something bigger and more serious, from a sinus infection to gastrointestinal problems.

If halitosis is stalking you, try these basic steps to freshen up:

- Drink plenty of water throughout the day.

- Eat balanced meals at regular intervals.

- Nibble on fresh mint or parsley in between meals.

- Brush your teeth twice daily.

- Clean your tongue, and floss between your teeth every day.

But if bad breath persists, have a chat with your dentist and doctor to rule out underlying issues and come up with a treatment plan.

Put Your Smile On

I don't know about you, but I always feel best with a smile on my face. And since I plan to be smiling for a very long time, I want my grin to be ready to gleam! Having a beautiful, sunny smile is so much easier and affordable than it used to be. We have a lot more information and a bevy of products at our fingertips to help us have—and keep—healthy gums and teeth at any age. One of the best decisions I ever made was having a good, long chat with my dentist about the small steps I could take to improve the look of my smile . . . and I've been beaming ever since.

10 Small Steps to a Supersexy Smile

❶ Eat well every day, with lots of fresh veggies and fruits and very few processed carbs.

❷ Drink plenty of water, to promote saliva production.

❸ Rinse your mouth with water after eating or drinking dark-colored foods or beverages.

❹ Scrape your tongue once a day.

❺ Floss daily before brushing.

❻ Brush at least twice a day for two minutes at a time.

❼ See your dentist at least twice a year for a cleaning and checkup.

❽ Get any medically necessary dental work done as soon as possible.

❾ Whiten your teeth if you want—but only with FDA-approved products and no more than once a year.

❿ Don't smoke.

A Sparkling Smile

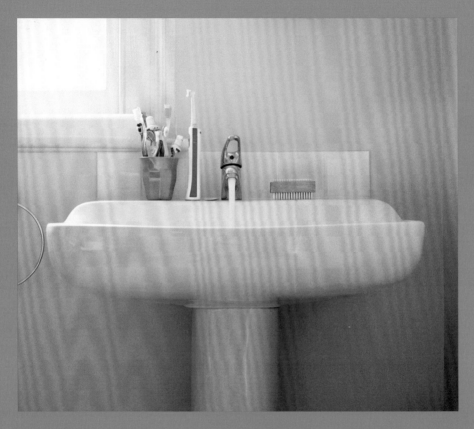

A few supereasy lifestyle changes will boost your smile to its brightest:

INSTEAD OF EATING WHITE FOODS,

Cut the carbs. To reduce cavities, stick to whole grains, veggies, and lean proteins. And although fruit is a healthy source of energy, it's also high in sugar, so opt for fresh fruit, not dried varieties, which are typically prepared with added sugars.

INSTEAD OF SUGARY CEREAL OR PASTRIES,

Start your day with yogurt. This delicious, healthy food (especially the plain or Greek varieties) offers a lot of benefits—one of which is keeping your gums healthy. The probiotics that occur naturally in yogurt may also help fight cavity-causing bacteria in your mouth. Steer clear of those with added sweeteners and, instead, mix in blueberries or strawberries for a satisfying, healthy breakfast.

INSTEAD OF GIVING UP RED WINE,

Follow it with a water chaser. To enjoy a glass of wine without staining your teeth, you could choose white, rosé, champagne or—my favorite—prosecco. However, if you're set on a heart-healthy red, just keep a glass of water nearby. Follow each drink of wine with a sip of water and discreetly swish before you swallow. This trick works for any dark drink, including coffee, black tea, grape juice, or cola. (But why are you still drinking cola?!)

INSTEAD OF DRINKING DIET SODA,

Drink water. Diet soda is terrible for your teeth. Sure, it's sugar-free, but it's also highly acidic and it can erode tooth enamel. As tough as it might be, it's best to wean yourself off sodas altogether—including diet. Swap them out for iced herbal tea or sparkling water. Your body and teeth will thank you.

INSTEAD OF BRUSHING WHEN YOU'RE ON THE RUN,

Eat an apple. If you can't brush your teeth after a meal, grab an apple (also known as nature's toothbrush), a pear, or some raw carrots, and munch away. While these crunchy treats do contain sugar, they can quickly trigger the saliva that will cleanse your mouth. Follow up with a few swishes of water.

INSTEAD OF TREATING YOUR TOOTHBRUSH LIKE A FAMILY HEIRLOOM,

Chuck it after three months—and sooner if you've been sick. To limit the growth of bacteria, consider keeping your toothbrush head in a cup of Listerine (the old-fashioned kind) when not in use.

INSTEAD OF USING MOUTHWASH FOR BAD BREATH,

Rinse with water and nibble on mint or parsley. Most mouthwashes have too much alcohol, which can dry out your mouth and actually make it more susceptible to bacteria and bad breath. Instead, keep your saliva production high and your breath naturally clean by sipping water throughout the day. Tuck a little bag of fresh mint or parsley leaves in your purse, and chew the herbs to brighten your breath anytime. Scraping your tongue in the morning helps, too.

INSTEAD OF USING YOUR TEETH AS PORTABLE PLIERS,

Treat them with respect! Don't chomp down on ice cubes or anything else that might chip or crack enamel or veneers. Treat your teeth with love and care, and they'll be with you for many years to come.

INSTEAD OF SMOKING,

Quit. In addition to all the other negatives, including an increased risk for oral cancers, smoking can cause teeth to yellow, and contributes to gum disease. And women who smoke have many more wrinkles around their lips, too.

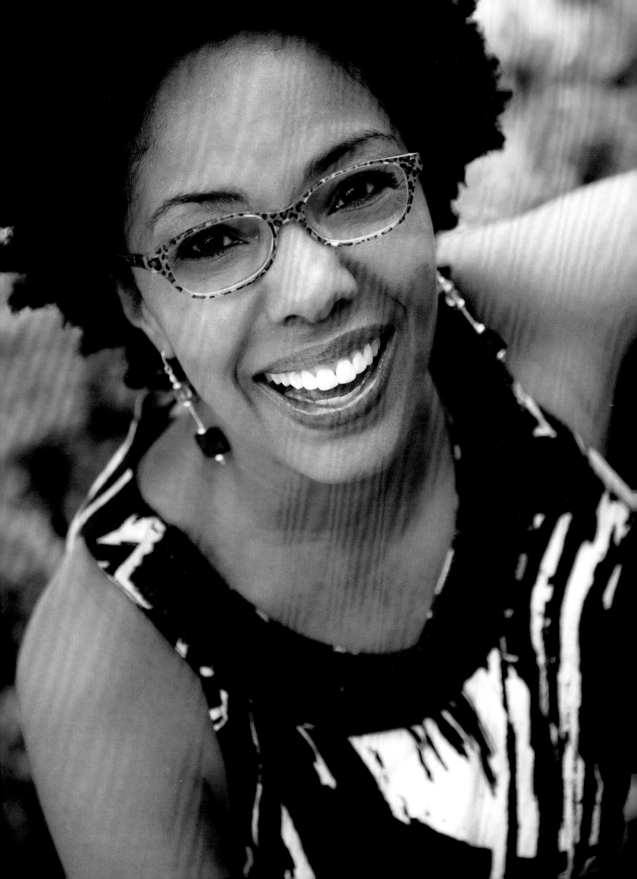

CHAPTER 9

Seeing Is Believing

"When a woman is talking to you, listen to what she says with her eyes."

—VICTOR HUGO

I'll never forget the day my eyes finally demanded the attention I hadn't been giving them. Prior to that moment I had no need to worry about my eyesight. I'd enjoyed 20/20 vision my whole life. No glasses. No contacts. No squinting. No nothing.

Well, that's a half-truth. I'd been ignoring several signs of what was coming down the pike. When I was 40, I noticed that the small print on labels was maybe less than crystal clear. By 42, anything closer than arm's length seemed a bit fuzzy.

But the day of reckoning arrived when I was 45. Preparing for a much anticipated trip to Tuscany, I bought an Italian-English pocket dictionary (complete with teeny-tiny print) and immediately started looking up the words for "hello," "goodbye," and "more wine, please." I think every one of my crow's-feet had its origins on that day. I squinted so hard my eyes were nearly shut.

That fateful day marked a series of firsts. I walked to my local pharmacy, bought my first pair of readers—and my first eye cream—then went home to make my first appointment with an ophthalmologist. And I appropriated my mother's 5x magnifying mirror (my first, her fifth).

I never looked back.

Eyes are our windows to the world and (as the saying goes) the windows to our soul. Through these lenses, we capture billions of images (and memories) over a lifetime.

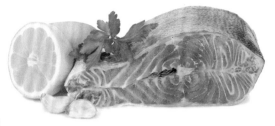

And yet most of us take our eyes for granted. According to a study conducted by the CDC, fewer than half of us contact an eye doctor even after exhibiting signs of vision problems or knowing that we're at high risk for vision issues. And as we get older, the likelihood of having problems with our eyesight increases—especially if we also experience common health concerns such as diabetes and hypertension.

How Our Eyes Change Over Time

As we celebrate each birthday, our eyes are aging right along with the rest of our body. Most of these changes are pretty normal:

- Eyelid muscles weaken, causing upper lids to droop.

- The skin under our eyes gets thinner, causing lower lids to sag and making the blood vessels underneath more obvious. If you're already prone to undereye circles due to genetics or allergies, they may become more pronounced.

- Eyelashes and eyebrows become more sparse. *(See page 206 for tips on how to fix this oh-so-common beauty bummer.)*

Eye Am So Glad to Know This

- Normal vision—usually referred to as 20/20—means that a person can easily read a vision chart from 20 feet away with one eye at a time.

- Oily fish—like salmon—help preserve good eyesight.

- Eyes can get sunburned.

- For most people, signs that reading glasses are in your future show up between ages 40 and 50.

- Eyes heal themselves quickly after getting poked or scratched.

- 80 percent of our memories are determined by what we see.

- Skin around our eyes is six to 10 times thinner than other facial skin.

- About 61 million adults in the United States are at high risk for serious vision loss, but only half have visited an eye doctor in the past year.

• Tear production slows down, contributing to dry, irritated eyes.

• Eyes may also tear up more frequently in an attempt to counter the dryness.

• The whites of your eyes may become more yellow.

• Your corneas can develop a whitish ring around the edge.

• The lenses of your eyes harden, leading to presbyopia, which makes it more difficult to focus on things that are close up. Yes, it's time to grab those reading glasses!

The Big Four

Although sagging eyelids and presbyopia are annoying, time can pose much more serious threats to your eyes. More than 3.4 million Americans over 40 are legally blind, and 17 percent of Americans have vision problems. By the time we reach 80, more than half of us will have developed at least one cataract. Cataracts, glaucoma, macular degeneration, and diabetes are among the most serious threats to your vision. They each have different causes but all share a common trait: They occur as you age.

CATARACTS

What they are: The proteins inside the lens of your eye begin to clump together, gradually blurring your vision until it's like looking through a waterfall. Some cataracts are barely noticeable and might not grow much at all. But left untreated, many cataracts can significantly impair vision, even though they are the #1 preventable cause of blindness in the world.

Watch for: Cloudy or double vision, increased sensitivity to glare, or seeing halos around lights. Some cataracts make colors appear less vivid.

Nag Alert! Vision Edition

You already know this but ...

• Don't share your mascara, eye shadow, or liner with *anyone*.

• Replace your mascara tube and brush every three months.

• Clean your eyelash curler of gunk and germs regularly. (Wipe with makeup remover and dry well.)

• Always, always protect your eyes from the sun and wind with sunglasses.

• Use safety glasses if you're working with tools or anything that might scratch, poke, or irritate your eyes.

> ## "The soul, fortunately, has an interpreter—often an unconscious, but still a truthful interpreter—in the eye."
> —CHARLOTTE BRONTË

Risk factors: Cataracts are caused by age and family history, combined with too much exposure to the sun's UV rays. But most of us will get at least one if we live long enough. While you could develop cataracts at any age, they tend to cause more vision problems after 60. Diabetes, smoking, obesity, high blood pressure, heavy drinking, and injury to the eye can all increase the risk of cataracts.

Treatment: The only cure for cataracts is surgery to replace the clouded lens with a clear artificial lens. More than three million cataract surgeries are performed every year in the United States. There are many lens options, including some that can also correct other vision problems, like astigmatism. Cataract surgery is an outpatient procedure performed by a cataract surgeon; it is effective in improving vision for 90 percent of people who have it. Also, while cataracts tend to worsen over time, most don't need to be removed unless they get big enough to impact your everyday activities. Your eye doctor should be aware of and monitor any problems. If you have cataracts in both eyes, surgery is usually performed on only one eye at a time, a few weeks apart.

AGE-RELATED MACULAR DEGENERATION (AMD)

What it is: The macula is the most sensitive part of the retina and is responsible for seeing things straight ahead of us. As we age, several different factors can cause the maculae to break down, resulting in partial or total loss of direct vision. In the most common, "dry" type of AMD, the retinal tissue becomes increasingly thin and fragile and may accumulate clumps of waste known as drusen. In the less common, "wet" AMD, abnormally weak blood vessels may grow behind the retina, leaking blood and fluids that can scar the retina and prevent the macula from functioning.

Watch for: There are no symptoms in the early stages, but an eye doctor may be able to spot drusen or unusual fluid deposits around the retina before any symptoms develop. If AMD progresses, it can cause blurred or distorted vision, or even a blank or gray area in the center of the visual field.

Risk factors: The causes of AMD are complex and not completely understood. However, smokers have double the risk of nonsmokers for developing

Floaters and Twitches and Redness—What Fun!

Is there no end to the jokes our eyes play on us? These little nuisances aren't usually serious, but definitely keep an eye on them (pun intended).

• **Floaters.** If you see a couple of small black dots or cobweb shapes in front of your eyes once in a while, don't be alarmed. These little clusters of cells or proteins are called floaters because they are literally floating through the middle part of your eyeball, casting a shadow on your retina. Most are annoying but harmless and often disappear over time, but check with your doctor if several new ones pop up suddenly, which could indicate a tear in the retina. If you have an ordinary floater that's obstructing your vision, try moving your eyes up and down and side to side to shift it out of your way.

• **Twitches.** Have you ever been totally engrossed in a good book when all of a sudden your eye starts to twitch? Annoying as it is, it's a fairly common occurrence. Stress seems to be the cause for most eye twitches. Other causes can be excessive crying, caffeine, fatigue, or an acute emotional event. If the twitching is chronic or severe, talk to your doctor about Botox, which can be used to temporarily "freeze" the muscle.

• **Redness.** There are many reasons why eyes can get red, including allergies, infection, dry eye, and inflammation. Thankfully, most can be treated easily. A trip to your eye doctor will help determine the cause and solution. Call your doctor immediately, however, if the redness is sudden and accompanied by pain.

AMD. Having high blood pressure or untreated heart disease also increases the risk, as does carrying extra weight around the abdomen and excess sun exposure without UV protection. AMD runs in families, and white people develop AMD more often than other races. Risk also increases with age—people over 75 have a 30 percent chance of developing AMD. Since women live longer, we get AMD more often than men.

Treatment: Wet AMD, which progresses more quickly, can usually be slowed with laser treatment and drugs, including some that are injected directly into the eye. The best treatment for dry AMD is a diet rich in dark leafy greens, fish, and high doses of vitamins C and E and beta carotene. If dry AMD progresses, taking nutritional supplements has been shown to be effective in preserving vision, but consult with your ophthalmologist for specific recommendations.

One More to Know: AION

This is a mouthful: Anterior ischemic optic neuropathy (AION) is a condition that causes partial or total blindness, most often in people over 50. While not common, it is serious, as vision loss is usually permanent. Frequently caused by lack of blood flow to the optic nerve, doctors call AION a "stroke of the eye."

Watch for: A sudden decrease in vision in just one eye, especially in the central or upper part of your gaze. Contact your ophthalmologist immediately if you experience any sudden change in vision.

Risk factors: The causes are not completely known and may be related to the natural shape of certain people's optic nerve. But people who smoke or have diabetes or high blood pressure appear to be at higher risk. AION can also occur after a sudden drop in blood pressure, such as after blood loss due to an operation or accident.

Treatment: If AION is suspected, your PCP will work with you to make sure your blood pressure is stable, and may order other diagnostics such as an MRI. Vision may improve somewhat over time, but there is no known treatment that will completely restore lost vision. Taking a low-dose aspirin daily may reduce the risk of a recurrence.

RETINOPATHY AND DIABETIC RETINOPATHY

What it is: Chronically high blood sugar levels can cause the tiny blood vessels in the retinas to leak blood and other fluids, leading to distorted vision. If not treated, retinopathy can lead to retinal scarring, retinal detachment, and even blindness. It is a common secondary illness for diabetics, but it is also possible to develop retinopathy without having diabetes.

Watch for: In early stages, you won't notice any signs of retinopathy without an eye exam. In fact, diabetes itself is often first detected by eye doctors. If left untreated, you may see floating spots that might disappear then recur, eventually limiting your vision. Early detection is critical to preserving vision, so get your eyes tested regularly no matter your health status, and at least once a year if you have type 1 or type 2 diabetes.

Risk factors: Having high blood sugar, diabetes, or prediabetes, having uncontrolled high blood pressure, or smoking. People who keep their blood sugar levels in the normal range cut their risk for diabetic retinopathy by 75 percent.

Treatment: Preventing and treating diabetic retinopathy follow the same prescription: Keep blood sugar levels in check. Maintaining low blood pressure and cholesterol may also help reduce the progression of retinopathy. If retinopathy develops enough to cause vision damage, drugs, laser treatment, or surgery may be needed, but early detection can reduce the risk of blindness by 95 percent.

GLAUCOMA

What it is: About two million Americans have glaucoma, a group of disorders that damage the optic nerve due to high blood pressure or increased pressure due to buildup of fluids in the eye. Just over 2 percent of Americans over 40 have glaucoma, but that percentage increases with age.

Watch for: Glaucoma is often overlooked because there is no pain and there are no symptoms in early stages, but it can be detected through regular vision screenings. If glaucoma progresses, it can cause diminishing peripheral vision and blind spots, and will slowly reduce vision.

Risk factors: Glaucoma tends to run in families; older people are more susceptible and blacks and Hispanics get glaucoma more often than non-Hispanic whites. However, the causes are not completely understood, and anyone could develop glaucoma.

Treatment: Topical drops are usually prescribed first, followed by oral medication if needed; surgery may be required if those options fail to stop the progression. Eyesight that is lost to glaucoma cannot be restored, but treatment may prevent further damage, so regular screenings and early treatment are essential.

THE TAKEAWAY?

The best way to keep from succumbing to any vision snatchers is to start having regular eye screenings at age 40. And you can greatly cut your risk for all the major eye diseases by protecting your eyes from UV rays, not smoking, keeping weight under control, and eating a healthy diet.

Know Your O's

There are three primary kinds of eye-care professionals, and it's important to understand the differences between them.

Ophthalmologists are true eye doctors. They are licensed medical physicians who specialize in the treatment and care of eyes and vision disorders. Ophthalmologists have attended medical school before training as eye specialists, so they are qualified to diagnose and treat all vision-related issues, and can perform surgery.

Optometrists are licensed eye-care providers who have a degree from an optometry college, but they are not medical doctors. They can perform basic eye exams to check visual acuity and prescribe corrective lenses and contacts but generally cannot diagnose or treat medical conditions or perform surgery.

Opticians are trained technicians who make corrective lenses according to the prescriptions issued by ophthalmologists and optometrists.

Many eye clinics employ all three "O's," and an optometrist can help manage garden-variety nearsightedness or farsightedness, and can update prescriptions for reading glasses. But for proper diagnosis and management of health-related eye issues, be sure to see an ophthalmologist regularly.

WHEN TO SEE THE EYE DOCTOR

Make an appointment with your ophthalmologist for regular checkups at least every three years starting at 40. After 55, make it every year.

Even if you have 20/20 vision right now, regular checkups are important. By starting to monitor your eyes before problems crop up, you'll have a baseline so that any changes are easy to detect. What's more, an ophthalmologist can often spot the early signs of other serious health problems, like high blood pressure or diabetes.

CALL AN OPHTHALMOLOGIST IMMEDIATELY IF:

• You lose all or part of your vision. This could be a sign of a serious condition, including an AION or a detached retina, either of which could lead to blindness.

• You see flashing lights or a cluster of little specks "floating" in front of your eyes. These may be symptoms of a detached retina or an ocular migraine.

• You have a sharp pain in or around your eyes. This could indicate a corneal abrasion or infection, which is a particular concern if you wear contact lenses.

When Drops Won't Do It

If you have persistently red, dry, or itchy eyes, it may indicate an underlying issue. Allergies, especially pollen allergies, are notorious for irritating eyes. If this is the case, then treating the allergy—with the advice of your PCP or an allergist—should resolve your eye trouble.

A second common culprit is a condition called blepharitis, which is an inflammation of the eyelid caused when tiny oil glands become infected or inflamed. While irritating, this condition doesn't usually cause any long-term problems. In addition to using moisturizing drops, consider two highly effective home remedies:

Hot compresses. Soak a fresh, clean washcloth in hot water and hold it to your eyelid for several minutes a few times a day.

Eyelid scrubs. Mix a few drops of baby shampoo with warm water, and gently wash the eyelid along the lash line, then rinse well.

If the irritation continues, check with your eye doctor.

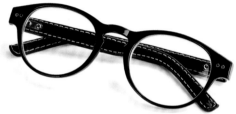

- You suddenly have blurred vision, tearing, redness, or a discharge from your eyes. Any of these could be the sign of an infection or allergy.

Welcome to the Specs Society

Whether you've worn corrective lenses since childhood or have just joined the presbyopia club, there are a few things you should probably know:

- Corrective lenses don't correct your eyes, just your vision. Put another way, glasses can't change the shape of your eyes, but they can change the shape of the images entering them, producing a clearer picture in your brain. There's a persistent myth that wearing glasses will further weaken your eyesight. Not true.

- As your eyes age, both near and distance vision may be reduced. You could use two sets of glasses—one for reading, one for driving—or you could opt for bifocal glasses, which are shaped to correct distance vision at the top and close-up vision at the bottom. Although traditional bifocals have a line across the middle, newer progressive lenses provide a seamless transition and look less aging.

- If you need glasses for both indoor and outdoor use but don't want a separate pair of prescription sunglasses, you can opt for photochromic lenses, which change from clear to dark as you go into sunlight. However, they do take a few minutes to transition completely and can be pricey.

You Should Be Framed

Eyeglasses have been trendy for several years now, and it's a great idea to treat your frames as part of your fashion statement. Even if you don't need corrective lenses, you should definitely be wearing sunglasses to prevent UV damage whenever you're outdoors during the day. So it's worth the effort to find frames that match your style and flatter your features.

As a rule, your glasses should complement your skin tone. If you have a cool complexion with blue or pink undertones, look for frames in black, silver, rose-brown, blue-gray, purple, plum, pink, jade, blue, and darker tortoise. If your complexion is warm, with a yellow or "peaches-and-cream" undertone, go for complementary camel, khaki, gold, copper, peach, orange, coral, off-white, fire-engine red, warm blue, or warm tortoise frames.

While many women choose neutral colors to match any outfit, don't feel that you have to limit yourself to black and tortoiseshell—or only one pair. Glasses come in a fabulous array of color combinations that can spice up your wardrobe. I have a small collection of readers in several shades of blue—my most flattering color.

Want Frames to Complement Your Face?

If your face is round, strong, angular shapes and dark colors are the perfect complement. Look for a frame that's wider than it is deep, and even try a pair with an upsweep at the corners.

If your face is oval, almost any style looks good on you, as long as it's not too big or too small for your proportions. Consider yourself lucky! Square and rectangular frames will work well, but don't be afraid to try other shapes, such as rounded or cat-eye styles, too.

So Your Vision Is Not What It Was ... Now What?

Just as we need to make adjustments to how we work out, what we eat, and how we care for our skin as we get older, so too must we adapt to changing vision. Here are some simple tips for dealing with this new reality:

• **Brighten up.** Improve the lighting in your home. Add extra lamps if possible, but even just swapping in brighter bulbs can reduce eyestrain.

• **Declutter.** The less clutter there is in your home, the easier it is to focus and the less likely you'll trip and fall over an item on a messy floor.

• **Spread the joy.** Leave a pair of inexpensive readers in every highly used room in your house, plus your car, office, and handbag.

• **Embrace technology.** Instead of squinting at print books, try a tablet device, which allows you to adjust the font size.

• **Magnify.** If you're struggling to see clearly when applying makeup or doing your hair, get a large magnifying mirror for your bathroom. These mirrors come in different strengths, so test a few to see what works best for you.

Your Eyesight Glossary

EYE ANATOMY 101:

CORNEA. The clear outer layer of the eye covering the iris.

IRIS. The colored membrane behind the cornea that opens and contracts to control the amount of light hitting the retina.

PUPIL. The dark center of the iris, where light and images pass through to the lens.

LENS. The clear structure behind the iris that changes shape to help you focus close up.

RETINA. A thin layer of nerves that lines the back of the eye and delivers the light impulses to the optic nerve.

OPTIC NERVE. The nerve that delivers impulses of light from the eyes to the brain, which translates them into images.

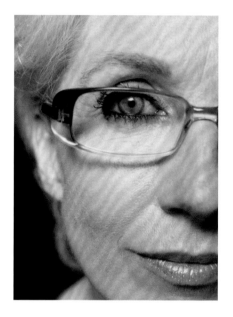

COMMON VISION PROBLEMS:

ASTIGMATISM. Blurry vision at all distances caused by an imperfect curve in either the lens or the cornea. Often noticeable in childhood but can usually be remedied through eyeglasses, contacts, or surgery.

HYPEROPIA. Also called farsightedness, it is a condition in which a person can see things clearly from a distance but less clearly close up. It's caused when the eye shape doesn't properly direct light onto the retina. It isn't the same as presbyopia *(see below),* which is age-related, although the symptoms are similar. Hyperopia can usually be remedied through eyeglasses, contacts, or surgery.

MYOPIA. This condition is usually called nearsightedness, because people with myopia can see clearly up close but have difficulty seeing objects far away, because the shape of their eyes focuses images too far in front of the retina. This common condition affects about one in four Americans and is often diagnosed during childhood but may worsen with age. It is usually remedied with eyeglasses, contacts, or surgery.

PRESBYOPIA. A natural consequence of aging, this progressive condition develops as the lens of the eye becomes less flexible and the eye can no longer focus to see close up.

TUNNEL VISION. A lack of peripheral vision, like wearing blinders. May be caused by glaucoma, eye strokes, detached retina, severe cataracts, or other eye disease, or may indicate other health conditions, especially if it appears suddenly.

If your face is square, oval or round shapes offer a pleasing contrast. If you prefer a rectangular frame, look for one with softened corners.

If your face is heart-shaped, consider a frame that balances the width of your face. Very light colors and materials, including rimless styles, will be especially flattering.

If your face is rectangular, try bigger rounded or curved frames to complement the longer lines of your forehead and jaw.

For sunglasses, larger frames mean more coverage and more UV protection for the delicate skin around your eyes. Consider wraparound styles for outdoor sports.

Going Frameless

About 80 percent of people over 40 who require corrective lenses opt for glasses. But contact lenses are a good option for many people and offer advantages like clearer vision and better peripheral sight lines. Plus they're easier to wear during exercise. Contacts can address a number of different vision problems, including nearsightedness, farsightedness, and astigmatism, and you can even get bifocal lenses.

But contacts aren't for everyone. Because they fit directly onto the surface of the eye, lenses can scratch the cornea, may lead to eye infections or protein buildup, and aren't recommended for anyone with severe allergies or dry eyes. Since the cornea has no blood supply, it needs to be exposed to the air to absorb oxygen, so contacts must be able to "breathe" enough to keep the cornea healthy.

Contact lenses come in two general types:

Soft lenses contain some water, which makes them somewhat flexible. They are more comfortable, but they don't usually last as long as hard lenses.

Contact Safety

The FDA has found that 40 to 90 percent of contact-lens wearers do not follow the proper procedures for wearing and cleaning their lenses, which means they are increasing their risk for permanent damage to their eyes and vision. So before you pop in your contacts, put on your backup glasses and read the fine print!

Hard lenses, or rigid gas-permeable lenses (RPGs), combine plastic with other materials that allow oxygen to pass through the lens. They offer very crisp vision, are more breathable, reduce the risk of dry eyes, and can last for up to two years or more with proper care. However, hard lenses can be difficult to get used to and usually cost more up front than soft lenses.

Most contacts of both types are "daily wear" and must be removed and disinfected at night, but some "extended-wear" options can be worn continuously for up to a week or more before cleaning. Some soft lenses, known as "disposable" lenses, aren't cleaned at all but must be replaced after a day, a week, or a month, depending on the variety.

Oh, and if you want colored contacts that enhance or change your natural eye color, the FDA says it's safe as long as you do it the right way: Get a prescription from a licensed ophthalmologist or optometrist, and order the lenses from a reputable manufacturer—preferably one recommended by your eye doctor—and carefully follow all safety recommendations. But never, never, never use lenses from a novelty, costume, or online store that doesn't require a prescription.

Regardless of what type of contacts you choose, you should always have a pair of backup glasses outfitted with your current prescription. You'll need them anytime you aren't wearing your contacts, lose your lenses, or develop an infection or other problem.

What About LASIK?

Sick of wearing contacts or glasses altogether? You may have another option to consider: One of the biggest breakthroughs in vision treatment in recent years has been laser-assisted in situ keratomileusis, much better known as LASIK, which was first approved by the FDA in 1998. This surgical treatment cuts away a small portion of the cornea in order to reshape it to better focus light on the retina.

LASIK is most commonly used to treat myopia, but can also help with hyperopia, presbyopia, and astigmatism. It is a fairly quick procedure that takes less than 30 minutes per eye and requires only local anesthesia. When successful, LASIK can reduce or eliminate the need for corrective lenses.

However, LASIK isn't for everyone. It can correct eyesight only within certain limits and can't necessarily provide 20/20 vision. Also, although it is a common procedure, there is usually discomfort afterward and there is a period of time when you will need to reduce your activities while your eyes heal. Like any surgery, LASIK comes with risks, which can include corneal infection or scarring, reduced ability to see color contrast, problems with night vision, and increased light sensitivity. Some people require follow-up surgery to achieve the desired results. In addition, many people still need reading glasses even after LASIK.

If you wear glasses or contacts and think you might be interested in LASIK, start by having a nice long chat with your ophthalmologist and, if you both agree that you're a good candidate, get recommendations for reputable and accredited LASIK practitioners. And definitely avoid any clinic that promises "20/20 vision" or claims that you'll never need glasses again.

Seeing Is Believing

Will I be throwing away my trusty 5x mirror anytime soon? Highly unlikely. In fact, I've upgraded to a 10x. But I'll keep up my vision-boosting habits for life.

10 Small Steps to Brighter Eyes

❶ Protect your eyes with sunglasses whenever you're outside.

❷ Eat plenty of dark leafy greens, orange vegetables, and fish.

❸ Keep your weight in check.

❹ Keep your blood pressure low.

❺ Avoid excess sugar and make sure your blood sugar stays at healthy levels.

❻ Get regular eye exams from a licensed ophthalmologist.

❼ Report any vision changes to your ophthalmologist ASAP.

❽ Wear corrective lenses as needed, and update your prescription regularly.

❾ Give eyes a rest from technology every 20 minutes or so.

❿ Ready? Say it with me: *Don't smoke!*

Bright, Beautiful Eyes

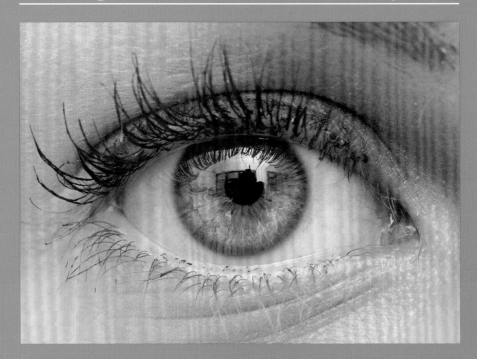

While the threats to our eyes range from the merely annoying to the potentially life-changing, we can keep most of them at bay by simply developing good vision habits. So in addition to making sure you have a regular date with an ophthalmologist, here are some actions you can take to keep your eyes young and healthy:

INSTEAD OF SMOKING,

Quit for good. Smoking is as bad for your eyes as it is for the rest of your body. It's been linked to an increased risk of almost all major threats to eyesight, including diabetes, glaucoma, and cataracts.

INSTEAD OF LEAVING YOUR EYES DEFENSELESS,

Wear sunglasses every day—rain or shine. Not only do they look cool, but sunglasses protect your eyes and the delicate skin around them from the elements. Make sure your sunnies block out 99 to 100 percent of both UVA and UVB radiation—this should be listed on the tag—and select an oversized or wraparound pair for extra coverage. A darker lens doesn't necessarily block more radiation, and if lenses are too dark you won't be able to see well. Choose gray, green, or brown lenses to see colors most accurately, and avoid red, blue, or purple tints, which can cause color distortion. Polarizing doesn't affect UV protection but can cut down on glare from water or snow, so it's a popular option for outdoor activities.

INSTEAD OF DEFAULTING TO THE SAME GLASSES FOR READING AND THE COMPUTER,

Try different strengths. Computer screens are usually farther away from our eyes than books or newspapers, so those of us with ordinary presbyopia generally need less help to make text and images legible. Whatever the strength of your reading glasses (1.50, 2.00, 2.50, etc.), try a pair half that number for computer work. Otherwise, you'll be making your eyes overcompensate, causing a different kind of eyestrain.

INSTEAD OF STARING AT SCREENS ALL DAY,

Give your eyes a rest. Almost all of us are spending more time using computers, tablets, and smartphones (often at the same time!). This can lead to eye fatigue, strain, and even dryness, because we forget to blink. Try the 20-20-20 rule: Every 20 minutes, look up from the screen and gaze at something at least 20 feet away (farther is better—like out a window) for 20 seconds. If you can't remember, try using phone apps like 20 Cubed or Eye Care to remind you. *Tip:* Get up and stretch or walk around at the same time.

INSTEAD OF GOING EYE TO EYE WITH YOUR COMPUTER,

Raise your seat. Another trick to combat screen-induced dry eye, is to raise your seat so you look slightly *down* at the computer screen, causing your eyelids to be more closed than open. This gives less room for air to circulate around your eyes.

INSTEAD OF USING DROPS TO GET RID OF THE RED,

Moisturize throughout the day. Dry eyes, which often result in bloodshot eyes, are especially common for women who have gone through menopause. However, simple over-the-counter moisturizing drops can easily relieve discomfort and refresh eyes. Be sure to choose a "lubricant" or "tears" type of moisturizer, and apply every few hours, all day. Avoid drops that claim to "get the red out," as they can create a rebound effect that leaves your eyes redder in the long run.

INSTEAD OF YO-YO DIETING,

Maintain a healthy weight. Being overweight or obese increases your risk of developing diabetes and other conditions that can result in loss of vision. If you are having trouble maintaining a healthy weight, talk to your doctor.

INSTEAD OF EATING JUNK FOODS AND EMPTY CALORIES,

Eat nutrient-dense foods. A diet rich in fruits and vegetables—especially dark leafy greens—is essential for eye health. Fatty fish, like tuna, salmon, and halibut, are loaded with omega-3 fatty acids, which studies show help to keep eyes young. Flaxseed oil is also a good source of omega-3s and may help to relieve dry eyes. And, of course, yellow and orange foods, like carrots, apricots, and sweet potatoes, are rich in beta-carotene, which gets converted into vitamin A—a famous eyesight aid.

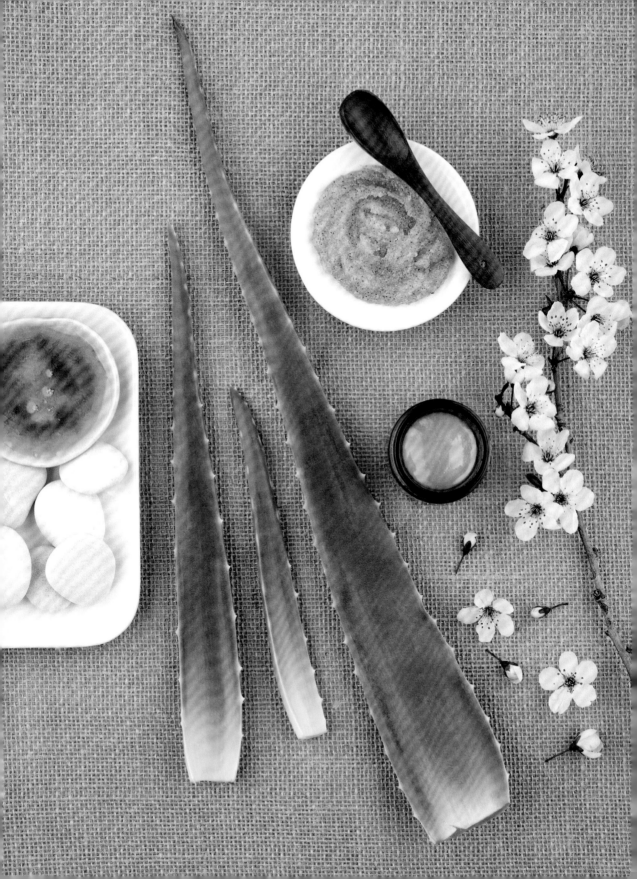

CHAPTER 10

Get Smart About Skin

"Nature gives you the face you have at twenty;
it is up to you to merit the face you have at fifty."

—COCO CHANEL

I was in my early 40s when I first noticed a real change in my skin—about the same time my eyesight started slipping. It surprised me to suddenly discover dark spots of pigment dotting my hands and little crinkles appearing around my eyes. In retrospect, of course, I should have realized that these "surprises" were actually the predictable results of years spent basking in the sun without sunscreen or hats (big mistake!).

The truth is, we don't always love our skin the way we should. In fact, we often abuse it, forgetting that skin is our body's largest organ and serves as the first line of defense against our environment. In fact, many of us have adopted some outright bad skin habits. I know I'm not alone in this, so raise your hand if you …

- Go to bed without removing makeup or washing your face—even just once in a while

- Think sunscreen is only for summer days at the beach

- Skip exfoliation

- Routinely dehydrate your body by drinking too much coffee or alcohol and not enough water

- Steam up your shower or bath with hot, hot water

> # 66 *Aging is a fact of life. Looking your age is not.*"
> —HOWARD MURAD

- Use the same skin routine you adopted when you were 20

- Overscrub, overpick, and undermoisturize

Sound familiar? Sadly, these mistakes will definitely take their toll. And when you throw lower levels of estrogen into the mix, you get what we might call a skin crisis: wrinkles, brown spots, redness, dryness, and more. But don't fret—because, as with any other habit … we can change.

Save Your Skin

Since skin care is an important concern for so many of us, I asked top dermatologists for their 10 best habits to help you take charge of your skin, starting now. They may help reverse some of the damage you've already done and will slow new signs of aging—so you can forge ahead with your best face forward!

❶ Wear sunscreen. This habit is #1 for a good reason: It works. Dermatologists all agree: The single most important thing you can do for your skin is to wear sunscreen with an SPF of 30 or higher every day, all year long. Apply it on all exposed areas, including your face, neck, chest, ears, and the tops of your hands. Even if you've already had a lot of skin damage from the sun (or, worse, tanning beds), using sun protection from now on will help your skin repair itself and prevent additional injury. Want to make it an easy habit? Choose a daily moisturizer with built-in sunscreen.

❷ Be sun-smart. Minimize your exposure to intense sunlight. If you're active outdoors, make sure you apply sunscreen, but also schedule outings to avoid midday sun, which is worst between 10 a.m. and 2 p.m. And always wear a hat, sunglasses, and sun-protective clothing. Wrinkles and brown spots are bad enough, but skin cancer is even more serious.

❸ Embrace exfoliation. Help your skin shed dead cells by gently exfoliating your whole body at least two to three times a week. You can use a special skin brush to help slough off dead cells before showering, or try this tip: Keep a jar of plain sugar in your shower, put a bit on your wet hands and gently massage all over. If you prefer a store-bought solution, you'll find a world of scrubs to try (Fresh's Brown Sugar Body Polish is a classic for a reason). To boost cell turnover on facial skin, use a mild exfoliant with either alpha hydroxy acid (AHA), for dry skin, or beta hydroxy acid (BHA), for oily skin.

❹ Moisturize. We lose moisture as we get older, so we need to replenish regularly—inside and out. When you get dehydrated, your skin does, too, leaving it dry, scaly, and wrinkled. Drink lots of water throughout the day and avoid excess caffeine and alcohol. Keep skin hydrated by applying moisturizer all over your body every morning and night. The best moisturizers combine humectants, like honey, aloe vera, glycerin, and hyaluronic acid—which draw moisture into skin—with occlusives, like shea butter and lanolin, which lock in that moisture. Another winning ingredient is ceramides, which is like the mortar that holds skin together. Some of my favorite everyday moisturizers are Olay Regenerist and CeraVe AM Facial Moisturizing Lotion with SPF 30.

❺ Use retinoids. Retinoid products, which are a form of vitamin A, work on the molecular level to help with skin cell turnover, boost collagen production, and thicken the skin. First introduced back in the 1970s to treat acne, they are also the best available treatment for reducing wrinkles and improving

The Most Common Skin Complaints After 40

- Dryness
- Fine lines
- Deeper wrinkles
- Sagging, especially around jawline
- Puffiness and dark circles under eyes
- Dark spots on face and hands
- Crepey skin

For the majority of us, our skin just gets drier and drier as we get older, especially after menopause. Our other skin problems are primarily caused by aging, genetics, lifestyle, and past sins (like sun worshipping and smoking). But most of these issues can be reduced—fairly simply—through better skin care.

sun- and age-damaged skin. The most powerful retinoids are available from dermatologists in very strong prescription formulas, like Retin-A and Tazorac. Lower-strength formulas with 0.5 to 2 percent retinoids can be purchased at drugstores and beauty stores, where they will be listed in the ingredients as "retinol" or as a "retinyl" compound. Great brands to look for are Neutrogena, Olay, and RoC. The OTC options are generally less expensive and easier to use but may take longer to show results. However, almost all formulas—prescription and OTC—will break down in sunlight and may make skin more sensitive to sun, so most should be applied only at night. Fair warning: Most women experience some irritation during the first few weeks after starting treatment, such as redness, burning, stinging, and peeling, especially when using prescription-strength products. Unless you have a truly terrible reaction, try to stick with it, because the irritation will subside and it can take several weeks to see results. If you've never used a retinoid before, start with one of the milder OTC versions and use it just two or three times a week before working up to stronger formulas. *Tip:* After washing your face, wait at least 10 minutes so skin dries before applying retinol, then add a bit of face cream over it if you need extra moisture.

❻ **Add antioxidants.** Much like antioxidants in food, antioxidants in skin care can reduce cell damage from free radicals, which break down cells and cause premature aging throughout the body. For this reason, most dermatologists recommend daily use of antioxidant serums, which are lightweight formulas that absorb quickly and penetrate deeply. For best antiaging effects, look for proven antioxidant ingredients, like vitamin C, green tea extract, grape seed extract, peptides, and niacinamide. A beauty industry favorite (and mine, too) is SkinCeuticals C E Ferulic combination antioxidant treatment. *Tip:* Wear it under your moisturizer.

❼ **Wash off makeup every single night.** I know, I know. You're tired. But makeup clogs pores, leading to pimples and blackheads and—possibly worse—it attracts free radicals, which can damage your skin as you sleep, contributing to wrinkles and premature aging. What's more, eye makeup can irritate your eyes and lead to infections. Gently massage face and eyes with a makeup remover that lifts dirt without irritating, like Albolene cream, and then tissue it off. Follow with a gentle facial wash appropriate for your skin. Even if you aren't wearing makeup, you should wash your face at night to remove sweat, dirt, and those dreaded free radicals. You might even consider investing in a battery-powered cleansing brush to deep-clean. Clarisonic is the leader of the pack, but Olay ProX makes a great one that isn't over-the-top expensive. Once you've slathered on a protective layer of moisturizer, your skin can actually heal itself while you sleep.

8 Keep your hands off your face. Think about everything you touch during the course of a day: food, money, cars, keyboards, and phones. Don't drag dirt and bacteria onto your skin, where it can cause all kinds of mayhem. Wash your hands throughout the day for good health (don't forget to moisturize afterward), but keep those paws away from your face.

9 See your dermatologist at least once a year. We all have different concerns, needs, and issues with our skin, ranging from wrinkles to spots to suspicious moles. Find a dermatologist you like and talk openly with her about what is going on with you so she can make recommendations that are right for your skin, not someone else's. Result? Your skin will look better, feel better, and age more gracefully.

10 Get regular facials. A professional facial by a licensed dermatologist or aesthetician is typically customized to your skin type and may include a deep cleanse with a steam treatment and mask, as well as a massage. Facials are great for unclogging and minimizing pores, increasing blood flow, and stimulating skin cell growth, leaving your skin glowing and radiant. In addition, seeing a skin-care expert regularly means you'll get up-to-date advice on the optimal home regimen for your specific needs. Get a facial once a month if you can, since the skin cell turnover is usually every 30 days or so, but at least once a season is a great way to help your skin adjust to changing weather conditions. If you have specific skin conditions, like oily skin or frequent breakouts, you might want to go more often.

Skin-Care Superstars

Every day there seems to be a new magic ingredient arriving on the market that promises to fix every skin-care issue you'll ever have. And while there will always be new developments in the science of beauty, here

are five tried-and-true powerhouse ingredients that really deliver the goods. Look for these in skin-care formulas:

Retinoids and retinol *(see Save Your Skin, page 176).* These #1 healthy skin tools can be used at prescription strength every night to build collagen, soften fine lines and wrinkles, thicken skin, and build skin strength. There are some new OTC retinol-based serums and eye creams that have been formulated for use during the day, but make sure you use sun protection on top.

Hyaluronic acid (HA). This powerful humectant is abundant in our skin when we're born, but it dramatically diminishes after 40, causing skin to lose moisture. To keep skin supple, hydrated, and plump as a baby's, look for HA in topical serums or moisturizers to improve elasticity and reverse free radical damage. It can also be used as a targeted wrinkle filler, in which case it is injected by a dermatologist to plump up skin.

Ceramides. These special lipid molecules occur naturally in the top layer of skin, where they act as a glue, sticking skin cells together and creating a protective barrier that plumps and hydrates skin. As an additive to OTC moisturizers, serums, and eye creams, ceramides help skin replenish the natural fats that we lose with age.

Peptides. Peptides are a type of amino acid found in the skin. While scientists are still arguing about exactly how peptides work, they seem to play a role in building collagen and retaining moisture. Skin-care products are often fortified with lab-derived peptides to help strengthen the skin and seal in moisture.

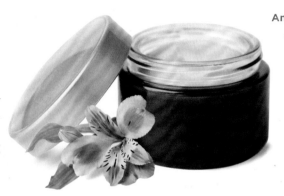

Antioxidants. When it comes to antioxidants, there's strength in numbers, so keep an eye out for formulas that include a combo. Vitamins C and E, coenzyme Q10, zinc, copper, green tea, and resveratrol are among the most potent antioxidants. All are known to fight free radicals—and premature aging—especially when combined.

A Potion Primer

Do you get a little dizzy standing in the health-and-beauty aisle these days? You're not alone. Here's a quick glossary to the terms you need to know:

SERUMS are lightweight liquids, usually water-based and often oil-free, that are used to deliver specific ingredients to your skin, where they will be absorbed quickly. Many include antioxidants, retinoids, or other skin rejuvenators.

MOISTURIZERS seal moisture into your skin and protect you from nasty things like pollution and free radicals. Heavier creams tend to have more oil, making them more moisturizing and better for dry skin, while lighter lotions with less oil are less likely to clog pores, making them a better choice for women with oily skin or acne. For daytime use, most of us do best with a relatively lightweight formula that allows us to apply sunscreen and makeup on top. Nighttime is perfect for richer, more hydrating treatments. Look for formulas that contain hyaluronic acid, ceramides, and niacinamide.

SUNSCREEN can be a separate product or may be incorporated into a moisturizer. Either way, check the label and be sure it includes two things: "broad-spectrum" coverage so it will protect you from both UVA and UVB ultraviolet light, and a sun protection factor (SPF) of at least 30, which blocks 97 percent of UVB rays. Sunscreens may use chemical UV absorbers, like PABA and oxybenzone, or mineral UV reflectors, like zinc oxide and titanium dioxide. *Tip:* Using makeup with added sunscreen is fine for bonus protection, but it isn't applied thickly or evenly enough to provide full coverage, so always use sunscreen or a sunscreen/moisturizer underneath.

EYE CREAMS are moisturizers specifically formulated for the delicate skin around the eyes, which tends to thin even more as we age. Look for formulas with things like caffeine or cucumber to reduce puffiness, Vitamin C and K to combat discoloration, and peptides to help plump up thin skin. Use eye cream during the day only, though. Even the best ones can seep into eyes as you sleep, causing puffiness and irritation. *Tip:* Keep your eye cream in the fridge for an extra cooling effect.

TARGETED WRINKLE FILLERS are fairly new to the antiaging lineup, but they can temporarily diminish the prominence of crow's-feet (though I prefer the term "laugh lines") and forehead furrows. There are two basic kinds: those with hyaluronic acid, which plump the skin to reduce wrinkles, and those with silicone or dimethicone, which sit on top of the skin to physically fill in wrinkles and make the surface of the skin look smoother.

Avoid Product Overload

It's true that our skin-care needs become more challenging as we age, thanks to all those years of mistreatment. But the answer isn't to pile on new treatments willy-nilly.

In fact, the best approach to skin care is a less-is-more philosophy, coupled with some strategic layering. Here's what to use and when:

NIGHTTIME

❶ **Makeup remover.** Use a nondrying makeup remover. Avoid those with alcohol in favor of nourishing ingredients, like oils or removers that specify "hydrating." Disposable makeup-remover cloths can be handy for travel, but many are too harsh for daily use, so approach them with caution.

❷ **Cleanser.** Wash with a mild cleansing oil or milk, which are generally better for dry skin than foaming cleansers. This will remove the last traces of makeup as well as sweat, dirt, and any residue from the makeup remover. Follow with a good rinse, and pat gently with a soft towel.

❸ **Retinoids.** Let skin dry for 10 minutes, then apply a pea-size amount of retinoid treatment all over your face and neck. Let it soak in for 15 minutes or so, then layer a light moisturizer on top. If you're just starting with retinoids, use them only two or three times a week until your skin adjusts. If you skip the retinol, apply a supermoisturizing night cream.

A Skin-Cancer Scare

I don't have many regrets, but here's a big one: For years I basked in the sun without protecting my pale skin. It wasn't until my 40s that I really started to take the "wear sunscreen every day" rule seriously. Result? Basal cell skin cancer on my chest when I was in my 50s. Luckily, my dermatologist spotted it during an annual skin exam and was able to remove it using Mohs surgery, the latest and currently best technique to remove skin cancer tiny layer by tiny layer, leaving as small a scar as possible. Lesson learned! I'm now a pro-sunscreen/anti-sunbathing advocate, and I'm here to tell you that it's never too late to protect your skin from the sun's dangerous rays.

> ## *The number of skin cancer cases due to tanning is higher than the number of lung cancer cases due to smoking."*
> —SKIN CANCER FOUNDATION

DAYTIME

Only women with oily skin (not too common after 45) need to wash with cleanser in the morning. For most of us, a nice splash of water is all you'll need to remove evening layers of treatments and creams. Twice a week, follow that with a gentle exfoliation. Rinse and pat dry.

Then, start layering your products, going from thin to thick.

❶ **Serum.** A good antioxidant serum can help smooth and brighten skin. With your face still slightly damp from your morning rinse, use a pea-size squirt of serum to lightly cover the entire face, then pat a few tiny dots of eye cream onto the undereye area, using your pinkie or ring finger, which are gentler than your index finger. Give that combo a few minutes to settle in and work its magic. (I like to do a few push-ups while I'm waiting for the serum to dry.)

❷ **Targeted wrinkle fillers (optional).** If you want to try them, they should be applied as a thin layer in the targeted areas only, and in between serum and moisturizer.

❸ **Moisturizer.** Apply a nickel-size amount of a good moisturizer to hydrate skin and seal in the first layers.

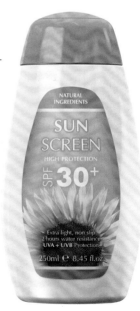

❹ Sun protection. If your moisturizer doesn't already have broad-spectrum SPF 30 in it, add SPF 30 sunscreen to your face before applying any makeup—and don't forget your neck, chest, the tops of your hands, and any other areas that will be exposed to the sun. For maximum effectiveness, apply chemical sunscreens at least 20 minutes before heading out the door. Mineral sunscreens are effective immediately.

❺ Makeup. Give your moisturizer and sunscreen a few minutes to soak in, then once your skin feels smooth and dry, apply your usual makeup.

Follow this simple program for a few weeks and you might find that you need less makeup—because your skin looks *that* good.

How to Do a Skin Self-Check

The American Academy of Dermatology has lots of great information and video tutorials on its website (*www.aad.org*) for monitoring your skin health, but the basic self-check is simple and easy to do before you hop in the shower. Make a habit of it!

• Take off all your clothes and stand in a well-lit room in front of a mirror. Use a hand mirror to help see your backside.

• Carefully examine the front of your entire body, then raise your arms one at a time and check out your right and left sides.

• Use the hand mirror to examine the back of your neck and part your hair to get a good look at your scalp. Yes, you can get skin cancer on your scalp—it's actually pretty common, especially along your part line.

• Next, look at your arms, hands, and palms—front and back.

• Then use the hand mirror to check out your back—and your butt!

• Last, look at your legs and feet, including between your toes and the soles of your feet.

Make a note of all the moles or spots you find so that you can easily tell if old ones change or new ones appear. If they do, or if you ever see any uneven moles, moles that have changed shape, scaly patches, strange bumps or sores, or skin that just doesn't look like the skin around it, get it checked out.

Healthy Skin Habits
You'll Wish You Knew 20 Years Ago

For a cool start to your day, dunk your face in a sink full of ice water. Hold it there for 30 seconds or longer, then do it two more times. Result? Radiant and glowing skin. *Bonus:* Some longevity experts claim an icy dunk helps build the immune system, too.

Use lukewarm water to wash your face and body. Hot water draws moisture out of your skin, drying it out. Instead, use the coolest water temperature that feels comfortable to you and finish a shower or face wash with a cool rinse to slow evaporation.

Use olive oil as a moisturizer. Olive and coconut oils are nonirritating and superhydrating for even the driest skin. They might be too heavy for facial skin but do wonders for arms, legs, elbows, and feet. Instead of body lotion, slather oil on after a shower while your skin is still damp, and let it soak in for a few minutes before dressing.

Pick up your product at the drugstore. While the fancy packaging on boutique brands looks pretty, there's no need to spend a lot on skin care. Many great products that include key ingredients such as hyaluronic acid, peptides, antioxidants, and sun protection can be found inexpensively at your local drugstore or at any mass-market retailer.

Choose a healthy glow over a sunny glow. Eat well, stay hydrated, keep your blood flowing—with exercise—and remember to exfoliate and moisturize. With these actions, you'll look radiant without creating more brown spots, wrinkles, and skin-cancer risk. If you simply must have color, get the look safely with tanning lotions that build a glow gradually, like Jergens Natural Glow or L'Oréal Paris Sublime Bronze Self-Tanning Serum (add a few drops to your regular moisturizer and watch the magic happen). The right makeup can also do the trick: Use a classic powder or cream bronzer on your face, or a tinted moisturizer one shade darker than your normal color.

Spread the love. Whatever you apply to your face is also important for your neck, chest, and the tops of your hands. That means retinol, moisturizer, and sunscreen.

Flip over. Sleeping on your stomach smashes your face into the pillow, adding to wrinkles. Try sleeping on your back (or at least your side) and invest in a silk pillowcase, which is more gentle on delicate facial skin than cotton.

The Skinny on Skin Cancer

While few of us are excited to see crow's-feet form, wrinkles really shouldn't be your biggest skin care concern as we age. What should? Skin cancer.

But skin cancer isn't all the same. Here's the rundown:

- Actinic keratoses are precancerous growths that appear as dry, scaly patches often found on the head, neck, hands, and arms. Left untreated, they can develop into squamous cell carcinoma, which is the second most common form of skin cancer.

ABCDE Spells Trouble

The American Academy of Dermatology and many other medical experts use this handy mnemonic to help you assess whether you're looking at an ordinary mole or a possible cancer.

A = asymmetry. Skin cancers are often irregularly shaped, unlike normal moles, which are usually even and round.

B = border. Normal moles typically have an even, well-defined edge. Cancerous moles often appear jagged, scalloped, or uneven.

C = color. Normal moles are a uniform color, but skin cancers often look splotchy and vary in color from one area to another.

D = diameter. If it's wider than a pencil eraser, be suspicious.

E = evolving. Watch for any mole or skin mark that is changing in size, shape, or color.

If you spot any of the ABCDE warning signs, call your dermatologist ASAP.

What About Botox?

Ah, yes. The not-so-secret secret of the stars (and lots of everyday people). Botox is made from an inert form of the toxin that causes botulism. When it is injected directly into the muscles of the face, it prevents them from contracting, reducing wrinkles and smoothing skin, particularly in the forehead and around the eyes and sometimes around the neck area too. Although it sounds scary, Botox is generally very safe, and results last for three to four months. While it can help soften wrinkles caused by sun damage, it won't help much with deeper wrinkles or plain old gravity. If there are lines and creases that bother you so much that they compromise your confidence, then ask your dermatologist whether Botox injections would be appropriate. Not everyone needs or wants them, but if you think the end result will bring you joy, then stop stressing and just go for it.

• Squamous cell carcinoma typically looks like a red bump, a scaly patch, or a sore that repeatedly reopens. Left untreated, it can spread to the surrounding skin and other parts of the body. It spreads faster than basal cell carcinoma but is less aggressive than melanoma.

• Basal cell carcinoma is the most common form of skin cancer. It usually looks like a flesh-colored bump or pink patch and, if not removed, it can spread to the surrounding tissue, including nerves and bones.

• Melanoma is the deadliest form of skin cancer. It frequently appears in an existing mole or as a new dark spot on the skin. Untreated, it can spread to other parts of the body, including lymph nodes. However, if caught and treated early, it has a high cure rate.

According to the American Academy of Dermatology (AAD), roughly two million Americans are diagnosed with a form of skin cancer every year, and it is the most common cancer in the country. As many as one in five Americans will develop some form of skin cancer, and about one in 50 Caucasians will develop melanoma. The rate is lower for African Americans (1 in 1,000) and Latinos (1 in 200). The good news? If skin cancer is caught and treated early, the survival rate is over 95 percent.

So the goal is to catch it early and treat it before it becomes dangerous. And, in most cases, that isn't so hard to do. Since we can see our skin, we can check it easily. Spend a few minutes every month doing a self-examination—and if you see anything unusual, call a dermatologist for a professional opinion.

Oh, and what causes skin cancer? By far, the single biggest culprit is too much UV exposure, whether from sunlight or tanning beds. Put on sunscreen every day and you cut your risk in half. Wear hats and protective clothing and stay out of direct sun between 10 a.m. and 2 p.m. and you cut it even more. And just say no to tanning beds, period.

Give Yourself a Hand

Hands have a way of looking way older than their years, and for good reason. Think of everything we put them through: scrubbing bathrooms, washing dishes, being exposed to sun and wind. Every minute of the day, moisture is being stripped away from our hands, leaving them dry, cracked, and crepey. Here are a few healthy hand habits to implement:

• Apply sunscreen to the tops of your hands every day.

• Wear gloves when washing dishes, loading the dishwasher, hand-washing laundry, or cleaning house.

• Keep mild moisturizing soaps by every sink, or look for nonsoap cleansers in the soap aisle. *Tip:* Although antibacterial soap sounds like a good idea, many studies have found that it doesn't prevent the spread of disease any better than regular soap and may be making bacteria more resistant to antibiotics! So skip the triclosan in favor of formulas with olive oil, aloe vera, or other moisturizing ingredients.

• Exfoliate your hands a couple of times a week along with the rest of your bod.

• Use hand cream after every time you wash your hands. Build collagen and skin thickness by choosing hand creams that contain hyaluronic acid and ceramides. (I keep CeraVe moisturizing lotion next to every sink in my house.) And pick up travel-size tubes to keep your handbag stocked.

• Slather on a superhydrating hand balm before bedtime. Look for formulas with serious moisturizers, like shea butter, or try straight olive or coconut oil. And if your mitts need extra pampering, slip a pair of lightweight cotton gloves on top to get a spa treatment while you sleep.

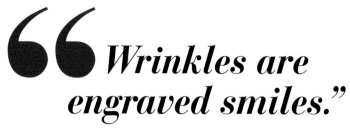

> ## *Wrinkles are engraved smiles."*
> —JULES RENARD

Creases and Spots and Wrinkles, Begone!

Unless you've been living under a rock (or an umbrella), chances are good that sun damage has left you with some lines and even a few brown spots (medically known as hyperpigmentation) on your face, hands, and other parts of your body. The good skin-care habits discussed above will help undo a lot of that damage, and if sun spots bother you, you can cover them with makeup. Some great products that give terrific coverage are Bobbi Brown's Retouching Face Pencil, Make Up For Ever's Ultra HD Concealer, and anything from Cover FX or Dermablend. Dab the product on the brown spot, then blend with your ring finger or a concealer brush.

However, if you want more rapid and dramatic results, make an appointment with your dermatologist to discuss the plethora of clinical treatments available to smooth skin and reduce discoloration:

Dermaplaning scrapes skin with a special dermatological razor, which improves skin texture, tone, and radiance—and removes peach fuzz, too! You can get a similar effect at home with devices like Dermaflash, but start with a professional treatment to make sure it's a good fit for your skin.

Dermabrasion uses a rotating device to literally sand off the outer layer of skin cells, reducing wrinkles and discoloration.

Fractional laser resurfacing helps remove the outer layer of skin cells and stimulate new cell growth to promote fresher, less damaged skin.

Intense pulsed light therapy is similar to laser treatment but uses pulses of light to stimulate collagen production and skin cell turnover with less peeling.

Hydroquinone bleaching creams are prescription formulas that chemically bleach skin to remove age spots or discoloration.

Photodynamic therapy is used to remove actinic keratoses but can also treat age spots by combining targeted light with a special cream that makes the light more powerful.

Trichloroacetic acid (TCA) or phenol peels use chemicals to remove the outer layer of skin, reducing wrinkles and discoloration.

All of these interventions can help with wrinkles as well as sun spots, but they may cause temporary redness, peeling, and other complications, so be sure you understand all of the risks as well as the benefits, and take recovery time into consideration before scheduling.

In addition, daily use of retinol helps reduce both wrinkles and sun spots. But for goodness' sake, slap on the sunscreen from now on!

The Skin You're In

As the place where your body meets the outside world, your skin is naturally going to reflect the years you've lived. While you might not love every mark of those years, embracing healthy skin habits will help stop the damage (and even reverse a lot of it), as well as lower your risk of skin cancer.

10 Small Steps to Sensational Skin

❶ Wear sunscreen every day—from head to toe.

❷ Stay hydrated with plenty of water and not too much caffeine or alcohol.

❸ Cleanse skin every night with a gentle soap.

❹ Exfoliate your face, hands, and body at least twice a week.

❺ Moisturize, moisturize, moisturize.

❻ Add retinoids, antioxidants, and other skin boosters to your routine.

❼ Protect skin from additional damage with proper clothing, gloves, hats, and sunglasses.

❽ Do a skin check every month and keep track of any changes you see.

❾ Visit a dermatologist once a year.

❿ Welcome the laugh lines: They're the signs of a life well lived.

Stunning Skin

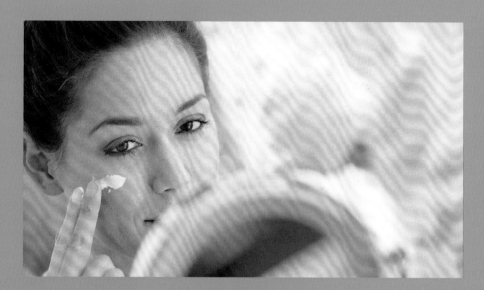

INSTEAD OF GOING UNDER THE KNIFE TO LOOK YOUNGER,

Do less to get more. Taking drastic measures to rework your face is a dated approach that will age you faster than any wrinkle. The more modern look is "less is more." There are many FDA-approved treatments that help plump, smooth, and improve the texture of skin. Work with a board-certified aesthetic dermatologist to review skin treatments like fillers, laser resurfacing, and dermabrasion, which can minimize or even reverse signs of damage and premature aging—all without surgery.

INSTEAD OF FOCUSING ONLY ON YOUR FACE,

Show some love to the skin below the chin, too. All the recommendations for your face apply to the rest of your body as well: Exfoliate, moisturize, keep shower temperatures low, and use sunscreen.

INSTEAD OF "YOUNGER,"

Think "better." We all need to get real when it comes to aging, and aim for looking better, not younger. If you adopt good habits and use treatments and procedures that improve your skin's health, texture, and tone, you might look a few years younger—but that should never be the goal, just a bonus. If "younger" is what you're trying to achieve, you're setting yourself up for disappointment. But if you aim for "better," then you'll take good care of yourself—which is almost guaranteed to show.

INSTEAD OF WAITING TO START A HEALTHIER ROUTINE,

Start today. It's never too soon to start taking good care of your skin.

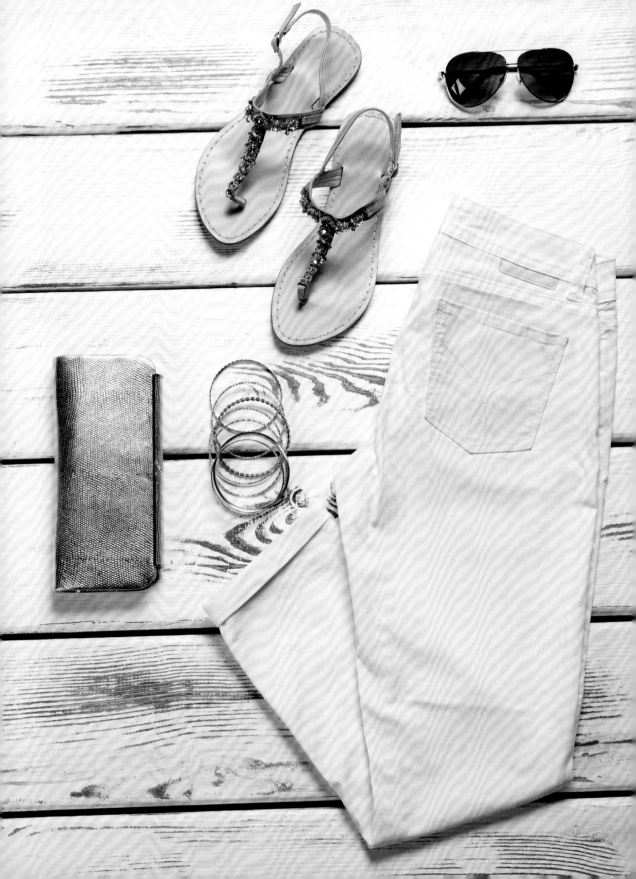

CHAPTER 11

Look the Part

"Always be a first-rate version of yourself,
instead of a second-rate version of somebody else."

—JUDY GARLAND

Something magical happens when you take control of your life. You walk taller, sit straighter, smile more, brim with energy, and—possibly most important—you sparkle with newfound (or refound) confidence.

That confidence may not always stay rock-solid, no matter how many push-ups you do or kale smoothies you drink. It will ebb and flow along with life's tides. But owning your power is essential as you take on all the new challenges and opportunities that lie ahead.

So whenever your self-assurance needs a boost, try this: In her must-see TED Talk, Harvard social psychologist Amy Cuddy says we can trick everyone—including ourselves—into believing we're ready to rule the world simply by looking that way. As she explains: "Our bodies change our minds, and our minds can change our behavior, and our behavior can change our outcomes."

So how do we do that? With one easy habit Cuddy says will put you on the road to confidence almost immediately: Stand as tall as you can, chin lifted, shoulders wide … and smile. Her research has found that making your body big and your attitude open can actually increase levels of testosterone—the confidence hormone—and decrease cortisol, the stress hormone.

Sounds too simple to work, you say? Well, guess what? It does! In fact, it's never let me down. I used to call it my "personal power pose," something I could use to boost my confidence whenever I felt anxious or low-energy. But after a few years of practice, I do my power pose just about all day long. Result? It's no longer a "pose." It's who I am.

Or, as Cuddy might say: "Do the Wonder Woman" and you'll become Wonder Woman!

Power From the Outside In

Even when you're standing tall and feeling great, you might still have days when the mirror doesn't quite reflect your inner glow. If there's a mismatch between your inner and outer selves, it can hobble your confidence the way too-tight shoes can keep you from running your fastest—whether after an archvillain or toward an elevator.

So if you feel like you've outgrown your wardrobe or like your old reliable beauty routine isn't working for you anymore, don't fret. A few simple changes can help you reclaim your inner warrior princess.

Let's take it from the top.

Glorify Your Crowning Glory

Not loving your locks? You're not alone. Most of us see big differences in our hair as we get older. The most common?

- Hair becomes more dry.

- Things get thinner on top.

- Grays starting elbowing their way through.

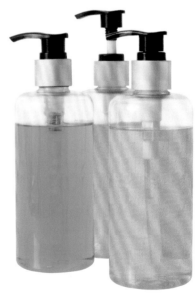

Add in a few decades of chemical treatments, overwashing, underconditioning, and blow-drying and you might not even recognize your poor hair anymore. (I used to describe my mop as "road kill on top of my head.")

Solution? Swap out yesterday's routines for new habits that will help the hair you have today.

Shampoo less. Most of us overdo both how often and how vigorously we wash our hair. Shampoo is very drying and strips the natural oils from hair, when what you really want—especially after menopause—is more moisture. You can rinse your hair every day (especially if you exercise) but limit shampoo to twice a week, and wash with conditioner alone on other days— it really works! On days you want to skip the water entirely, spritz in a little dry shampoo to freshen up and absorb excess oil. But if your hair demands more frequent washing, use a dime-size amount of a moisturizing nonsulfate shampoo.

Cleanse your scalp only. Lather up your scalp, not your hair. Shampoo will get distributed through your hair as you rinse, cleaning on the way out, so don't worry about scrubbing throughout your hair. This will reduce shampoo's ultradrying effect on your locks.

Condition more. You might worry that conditioner will make your hair greasy, but it's the rare woman who has oily hair after 45. The reverse is more often the case: hair that's overprocessed and very dry. Pour that conditioner on. Want even more moisture? Work in a hair masque or some olive oil, cover with a shower cap or old tee, and let it soak in while you do housework or exercise, or try a leave-in conditioner. I always have something moisturizing in my hair when I run.

Let hair air-dry. Cut back on heat exposure from blow-dryers and curling irons—and the abrasion of terry-cloth towels. Instead, gently scrunch wet hair with a T-shirt or microfiber hair towel, apply styling product, and either allow your hair to fall naturally or position it with clips. Let it air-dry, then shake it out. In a rush and must dry your hair quickly? Let it air-dry for as long as possible, then finish with a diffuser and keep the blow-dryer on a low setting. If blow-drying is essential to you, just make sure to keep the heat setting low and avoid pulling hair too much with a brush to minimize damage.

Shun the sulfates. Sulfates are substances used to create suds in everything from shampoo to laundry detergent. However, they also tend to strip color from hair and make it drier and frizzier. While sulfates are common, especially in inexpensive shampoos, there are plenty of sulfate-free formulas to choose from at all price points, so read the ingredients before you buy.

Hold your style with dry shampoo. Hairspray is very drying and so old-fashioned. Ditch it in favor of this terrific trick from top hairstylists: Flip your head over, then spritz some dry shampoo close to your scalp and gently massage the shampoo onto your scalp and through your hair. Stand up and position hair, lifting hair at the roots with fingers. It's an especially effective way to plump up thinning hair. You can also spritz a little on your fingertips to smooth flyaways.

Use your fingers. Brushing can tug hair, break it, and make it frizzy. The best way to get knots out is to gently use your fingers, not a comb—and to do it in the shower while the conditioner is still in. Afterward, while your hair is damp, use your fingers, not a brush, to position it.

Get to the root of thinning hair. If your tresses are getting sparser, visit your dermatologist straightaway to figure out what's going on and how to fix it. If your hair is thinning at the roots, your doc can help you track down any medical causes. And don't wait! You may be able to slow or stop hair loss with prescription-strength minoxidil or an OTC version, like Rogaine, which is applied directly to the scalp to help repair injured follicles. But if your hair is thinning because it's breaking, then adopt the healthy habits in this chapter and be more gentle with your locks going forward, including looking for a pro stylist who specializes in hair that's thinning.

Let it be what it is. For decades I "blow-fried" my curly hair to make it straight. It was a revelation when I finally put away my blow-dryer and let my waves be free. Whatever your hair is—straight, curly, wavy, coarse, fine— find a stylist who will shape it to let the real you shine through. Spend some time looking through magazines and websites to find examples of women who have hair texture like yours to get a better idea of what cuts work best. Not only will you look better, you'll save time and money and avoid damage from styling.

Give flat hair a lift. After cleansing hair, flip your head over and add a bit of volumizing mousse to your roots. Flip hair back up, then fluff the top to add height and hold with a few hair clips. Let it air-dry or use a blow-dryer with a diffuser on a low setting. To finish, spritz some dry shampoo on your hands and gently place your fingers under your hair, close to the top, lifting everything up. No more flattop.

Choose Your Best Cut

For hair that suits you to a T, choose a style that flatters both your hair's natural texture and your face shape.

HAIR TYPE

CURLY, WAVY, OR THICK HAIR. Longer layers will maximize natural wave. Let hair air-dry to keep frizz to a minimum. *Translation:* Pick a style that doesn't require straightening.
STRAIGHT HAIR. Blunt cuts work well, as do bobs and lobs (longer, and sometimes layered, bobs). Straight hair looks great at any length, as long as ends are healthy, not straggly.
FINE HAIR. Shorter cuts keep extra weight from dragging fine hair down. A lob between the chin and shoulders is low-maintenance and sexy.

FACE SHAPE

ROUND FACES are complemented by long layers, uneven cuts, and bold elements, like wide bangs or a deep side part. Look for styles like pixies, which draw attention to your cheekbones, or long bobs, which create a vertical line to balance the fullness in your cheeks.
OVAL FACES look great with loose layers, especially those that start near the cheekbones. A center part—a look that can be a bit too severe for most women—can be a good option for this face shape, especially with a tousled do. But also try boldly side-swept or blunt-cut bangs.
SQUARE FACES pair well with cuts featuring softly textured ends, whether in a short tapered bob or a shoulder-length shag. Long hair with an off-center part also looks great, whether straight and sleek or textured for loose waves that start below the jawline.
HEART-SHAPED FACES are nicely balanced by bobs that end just below the jawline, shoulder-length or pixie cuts with deep side parts, and long hair with more fullness below the ears than on top.
RECTANGULAR FACES are flattered with chin-length bobs or A-line lobs. Shoulder-length or longer hair can look great, too, especially with some waves or fullness around the face. Layered bangs and side parts, which add a soft horizontal element, are great for balancing the length of your face.

A PARTING THOUGHT

Finding the most flattering part for your face shape can take a little experimentation. While some women love center parts, they can be aging and a bit harsh on many of us. Side parts or bangs are usually more flattering, softer, and modern. But if your preference (or your hair's natural inclination) is to part in the middle, try a zigzag part or go a little off-center.

Don't be afraid to let it flow. There's a tired old notion that long hair is only for young women. But celebrated hair stylist Frédéric Fekkai says that's all wrong. Your ideal hair length and style depends on your lifestyle, personality, height, silhouette, and the health of your hair. If it's brittle and damaged, then chop it. But long, healthy locks on a woman of any age can be beautiful and very sexy. Just don't let it overwhelm you. As Fekkai points out, long works best if it's not too long for your proportions.

Eat more eggs. For stronger hair, eat more eggs, which offer a powerful combo of iron, biotin, and lots of protein. Pomegranates and any foods rich in omega-3s, like salmon, avocados, olive oil, and pumpkin seeds, also work hair wonders.

Think contrast. Hair in a single block of color actually makes most women look older, not younger—especially if it's too dark or light (yes, you *can* be too blonde!). If you prefer single process to cover gray, find an experienced colorist who can weave in highlights to create contrast and depth, especially around your face.

And speaking of gray …

Go Gray the Right Way

Gray happens. As we get older, our follicles stop producing melanin, the pigment that also gives color to skin and eyes. At the same time, hair becomes more wiry, dry and—yep—thinner. So while getting the right cut and style is important at any age, it becomes even more essential once grays grow in.

In our youth-obsessed culture, it takes a badass woman to go gray all the way. But if you decide to take the leap, follow these simple steps to be a modern silver fox (or even partially silver, like me):

Mix it up. If you don't want to go completely gray but don't want to cover it completely either, opt for highlights and lowlights mixed with your gray. Pay special attention to warm highlights around your face and try a layered haircut to help it all blend harmoniously.

Ease into it. If you want to stop coloring entirely, transition into gray from single process by having your colorist weave in highlights and color fewer

> ## "Whether I'm wearing lots of makeup or no makeup, I'm always the same person inside."
> —LADY GAGA

and fewer sections as the months go by. Keep hair shorter to make the transition move more quickly.

See a pro first. Even if you're a dedicated DIY home colorist, consult with a pro who can show you how to work with your beautiful new gray as it comes in.

Cut it right. Get a great haircut that flaunts your new locks and cooperates with your hair's changing texture. Short edgy styles pair well with gray—think of actress Jamie Lee Curtis—but so do glamorous longer looks like those sported by model Carmen Dell'Orefice and musician Emmylou Harris. If your gray is still coming in, cropped hair can make uneven color look more uniform.

Shine on. There's no reason gray has to be gloomy. Use styling products that moisturize and add shine by smoothing on a light coat of argan oil or a similar lightweight product. *Tip:* Spritz just a bit of oil on your palms, rub to warm, flip your head, and fluff your hair with your hands. Avoid applying it to the roots, which can make it look greasy and weigh hair down.

Match your makeup. As your hair color changes, you may need to adjust your makeup, too. Depending on the undertones in your hair and skin, you might want to shift to warmer or cooler hues to make sure you still look vibrant, not washed-out. *Tip:* Red lips can be stunning and supersophisticated with gray or white hair.

Whether long, short, colored, or gray, embrace the hairstyle that makes you feel bold, beautiful, and bodacious. And remember this: You can always change it!

Makeup: The Transformative Power of "Up"

Makeup is a terrific tool to enhance your natural beauty—laugh lines and all. But for most of us, the products and techniques that worked so well just a few years ago are due for an update.

THE MOST COMMON BEAUTY CONCERNS

- Skin texture is changing, including fine lines, wrinkles, and enlarged pores.

- Discoloration, uneven tone, undereye circles, and brown spots are appearing.

- Eyebrows and eyelashes are getting sparser.

What Should You Look For at the Beauty Counter

If your old products aren't quite matching the face you have now, keep an eye out for replacements with these key words:

- **Moisturizers.** Even if you've upped your skin-care game to include more moisturizers, makeup formulas with added hydration are a boon, especially around lips and eyes. Look for products specifically marketed for dry skin and those that include peptides and hyaluronic acid.

- **Creamy formulas.** Creamy eye color and blush enhance skin and reduce fine lines and wrinkles—and they're easy to apply. Unless you have very oily skin, avoid matte finishes, which may end up looking dry and cakey.

- **Light diffusers.** An increasing number of beauty products feature ingredients known as light diffusers, which hide minor skin defects by reflecting light, to create the illusion of smoother skin. Light diffusers don't fill in lines or wrinkles, but they can make them less noticeable. Look for ingredients like crushed pearls, mica, or minerals like titanium dioxide—but avoid supersparkly formulas. The idea is to create a soft-focus look, not a glitter bomb.

- Lips are thinning, and the skin around them is getting creased.

- There is overall drooping, sagging, and puffiness (especially under eyes).

Good news: A few basic strategies and product swaps can address all of these concerns.

MODERN MAKEUP MANTRAS

As you review your beauty routine, consider these five tips from the pros:

Keep it light. Too much makeup can age you faster than none at all.

Brighter is often better. As we age and our natural coloring becomes a bit muted, lighter and brighter shades may be more flattering.

Dewy is good. Cakey or greasy is not.

Use makeup to enhance, not hide. Not only is confidence more attractive, but too much concealer and cover-up can often end up drawing more attention to your "flaws."

Healthy living is your best beauty secret, because all the makeup in the world can't help neglected skin.

Base Layers: A Bottom-Up Beauty Strategy

Your best look always starts with a clean, moisturized face. After that, consider these helpful products to boost your natural glow.

PRIMER

A relatively new category of makeup, primers go on first to smooth and conceal minor imperfections so that everything you put on top looks better and lasts longer—kind of like the Spanx of the cosmetics world. Good primers, like those from Laura Geller, MAC, and Smashbox, also even out skin tone and reduce the appearance of fine lines and pores—but none of them will fill in deeper wrinkles, no matter what the label claims.

FOUNDATION, TINTED MOISTURIZER, BB CREAM, OR CC CREAM

Any one of these can be applied on top of—or instead of—primer to even out skin tone and add dewiness. And that may be all you need for a fresh bare-faced look. *Tip:* Test the shade of your base layer by applying a small amount to the inside of your arm a couple of inches above your wrist, which is a close match to your facial skin. It should blend invisibly. If you have sensitive skin, that's also a good spot to do a patch test to see if a new product will cause a reaction.

The Concealer Cure

Do you want to hide your amazing face? Absolutely not. But there may be a feature or two you'd like to minimize. Enter one of the most useful tools in your makeup kit: concealer.

HOW TO CHOOSE THE RIGHT CONCEALER

Concealers come in different forms, including sticks, liquids, creams, and cream-to-powders. As a rule, cream and liquid formulas work best for most skin types—if you're careful not to cake it on. For undereye use, select a hydrating formula in a color one or two shades lighter than your natural skin tone, which will also work as a highlighter. For the rest of your face, a close match to your foundation is a better bet. The trick is to apply lightly and blend well. *Tip:* Don't use any concealer until you've applied your base. You might not need it after all!

WHAT CAN CONCEALER DO FOR YOU?

Reduce undereye shadows or bags. Whether it's due to genetics, thinning skin, allergies, or lack of sleep, we all have dark circles from time to time. Use your ring finger or a concealer brush to dab concealer just under the eye, then gently tap to blend. Magic! You can also try a brush-on highlighter that uses illuminating particles to camouflage the dark area. Remember that you only want to brighten the undereye enough to make it blend; if your concealer is too thick or too light-colored, it will actually draw more attention to the issue. Here's a trick from the pros: If you have bags or puffiness under your eyes, apply a little bit of lighter concealer *under,* not on, the puffy area.

Soften the nasolabial folds, aka "smile lines." With a small brush, lightly dab concealer slightly above the lines, starting from your nose and continuing down to the corner of your mouth. Then, using a cosmetic sponge, lightly tap the concealer until it blends in seamlessly.

Cover brown spots. To minimize dark spots, apply concealer that matches your skin color directly to the spot, then apply foundation around it. Using a flattop foundation brush, buff the foundation into your skin in a circular stippling motion, blending the edges without rubbing it all off. This works on the back of your hands, too.

Cover red areas around the nose. Dab concealer on lightly with a small concealer brush, then blend evenly.

Keep It Up!

As we get older, things start to drag down, thanks to lower estrogen, loss of collagen, and good old gravity. While a dedicated skin-care regimen is the most important way to keep your glow, you can also use the simple power of makeup to lift and brighten your whole face.

All About That Base

These days there are several types of base layers, and, while they all have similar functions, understanding the differences can help you choose the best product for your needs.

• **Foundation.** This makeup is designed to match your skin tone, provide a smooth base, and cover imperfections; foundation usually provides the most coverage of the bases. Look for sheer liquid or gel options and avoid "velvet" or "long-wearing" formulas, which tend to be thick and heavy. Don't cover every inch of your face. Use foundation only to even out discoloration.

• **Tinted moisturizer.** With just a bit of coverage built in, tinted moisturizers are lighter than foundation and might be better for extra-dry skin. Many contain sunscreen, too. You can make your own tinted moisturizer by blending your favorite foundation with your favorite moisturizer. Easy-peasy.

• **BB and CC creams.** "BB" stands for "blemish balm" or "beauty balm," while "CC" is short for "color and correct." These creams are about halfway between tinted moisturizers and foundation in terms of coverage but usually contain added products to help even out skin tone and treat specific skin concerns. CC creams are specifically designed to cover redness and usually provide more coverage than BB creams.

For an instant face-lift: Dab highlighter in three places: under your eyebrows, on the tops of your cheekbones, and on the inside corners of your eyes. Blend well. The net effect lifts (and lights!) everything up. Aim for a highlighter that's creamy and has a bit of shimmer (not sparkle!), like Benefit's High Beam, Boots No7 Skin Illuminator, or my personal favorite, Yves Saint Laurent Touche Éclat.

For serious uplift: Try contouring. It takes a little practice, but contouring is a fantastic way to define your features for photos or special events. The secret is to keep it light and well blended. To do it right, you'll need two concealers or foundations: one that's a shade or two lighter than your skin tone and another a shade or two darker. Some companies even make double-sided contouring sticks or palettes for this purpose. Cream formulas are easiest to blend, especially when applied with fingers. Choose colors that match the undertones in your skin and avoid orange or red tones in your shading color.

After applying your base layer, apply the darker shade in a short vertical stroke at each temple and the hollow of your cheeks, starting just below your cheekbones. To slim your nose, add a thin stripe of dark shading along each side. Conversely, if you want to create more roundness in your face, shade your hairline and the lower part of your chin. Then, using your fingers or a damp cosmetic sponge, tap over the contour color in small circles to blend.

Now it's time to make things pop! Apply the lighter shade along the tops of your cheekbones. Add a light layer above your brows, then one dot each in the center of your forehead, on your chin, and on the tip of your nose. If you want extra length, put a stripe down the bridge of your nose. And then blend, blend, blend until there are no visible edges between the concealers and your foundation. Dust with a translucent setting powder, and there you have it: beautifully defined features without overdone makeup. Or surgery.

Blush Boost

Often overlooked, blush brings life to your whole face. But avoid a harsh '80s-style streak along your cheekbones, which can make you look drawn and hollow. Instead, redirect the focus to the upper part of your face by using your fingers or a special brush to blend a touch of cream blush directly on the tops of your cheekbones and sweep up and out toward your hairline. *Tip:* Even if you've been a die-hard powder-blush lover your whole life, this might be a good time to give cream formulas a try.

They're easier to apply and more moisturizing for dry skin, and they don't settle into facial wrinkles and fine lines the way powders can. Plus you can quickly build up light layers, giving a much more natural glow.

Play Up Your Eyes

No matter their shape, size, or color, your eyes convey everything. So why not give them extra attention before heading out the door for work, play, or a big night out? A little makeup can do a whole lot when it comes to your eyes, providing an extra spark and reducing some of the less charming signs of aging.

EYEBROW GROOMERS

A strong brow is one of the best ways to give your face a visible lift. But while thinning or graying brows can be frustrating, brows that are obviously drawn on will make you look older than you are. For a natural brow, first remove any stray hairs with tweezers to keep your shape defined. Then, fill in sparse areas with a pigment that matches your brow color to create a soft natural-looking texture. Eyebrow pencils are easy to use, but if you have a steady hand, powders look even more natural and can be applied with a slightly damp brow brush or toothbrush. The key is to stroke in the same direction as your eyebrow hairs, using a short quick motion, and to build layers subtly. To keep the color in place all day, finish with a touch of a clear brow gel, which comes packaged like eyelash mascara.

EYE SHADOW

For everyday wear—and the most flattering look for most women—go for neutral eye shadow colors and keep it simple. Cream formulas add moisture and dewiness. Choose a matte shade close to your natural skin tone and apply it from the lash line to your brow bone using an eye shadow brush, or your finger for creams. Then apply a darker shade (brown or gray works well, as long as it's not too dark) in the area above the crease line on the lid. Blend and sweep the darker shade toward the outside corner of your eyes. This will give a subtle lift and move the focus up. For added emphasis, apply a slightly darker shade as close as you

For the Perfect Arch, Don't Go It Alone

Instead of shaping your eyebrows on your own, make an appointment with a brow specialist. This beauty expert can help you create the right brow shape for your face and teach you how to maintain it at home. Many salons and spas offer this service, or ask for recommendations at your favorite cosmetics department.

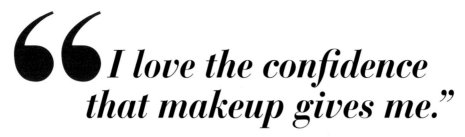

"*I love the confidence that makeup gives me.*"
—TYRA BANKS

can get to your upper lash line, using a flat-sided eyeliner brush. Start at the inner corner of your eyelid and work your way out. Your eyes will pop just a little more, yet still be very natural-looking.

EYELINER
Liner helps define eyes, and makes you appear more awake. To avoid dragging things down, apply it to your upper lids only, focusing on the outer corners. If you aren't using a shadow, first dust a bit of translucent pressed powder over your lids to absorb any excess moisture. Next, apply a pencil liner by dotting it between your upper lashes, then connect the dots with a tiny liner brush. For extra oomph, go over the same line using either a pen or gel liner. Or, for a softer look, smudge the line with a Q-tip, pinkie finger, or eyeliner brush. And choose your product carefully: Dark, heavy liner can make eyes look smaller and more tired. Try a superskinny felt liner in brown, charcoal, or navy, and follow the natural lash line to provide light, bright definition.

MASCARA
Skimpy stick-straight lashes can make you look tired, but full lashes add sparkle to your eyes and face. Curling your lashes before adding mascara makes them look even longer. Carefully clamp down on lashes with your eyelash curler, getting as close to the base of the lashes as you can without pinching the eyelid, and keep pumping the curler as you slowly move up and out to the tips.

Then, for the most uplifting look, wiggle a volumizing mascara onto your upper lashes only, starting at the roots and slowly stroking up and out through the ends. Let it dry, then add a second coat for extra volume. Avoid accenting the lower lashes, which can draw attention to dark circles and make your eyes look droopy.

Powder Less, Glow More
Powder is useful as a final layer for setting makeup, absorbing oil, and providing light coverage, but it can be drying and tends to magnify pores and imperfections,

making skin look older. Personally, I use powder only when I'm going to be on television or in photos. If you need it on the T-zone, try a translucent setting powder dusted lightly over the area with a loose brush. Or just use blotting paper to get rid of shine as needed.

Lipstick, a Love Story

Lipstick brightens your entire face, makes lips look fuller, and can even be used as blush in a pinch. True story: I love mine so much that if I leave home without it, I either go back for it or zip to a store and buy a new one. I even carry a tube in my running belt!

For maximum impact, look for creamy formulas that will show the texture of your lips while spotlighting some gorgeous color. Exfoliate first, then prep with a colorless lip liner, which will keep

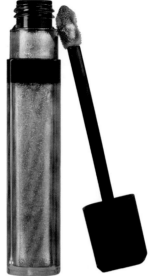

Secret Beauty Superheroes

These little helpers more than earn their keep.

• **Tweezers.** Tweezers are not only ideal for shaping eyebrows to perfection but also for keeping unwanted hairs off our chins—and elsewhere.

• **Pointed-tip cotton swabs.** These little problem solvers can remove nail polish from your cuticles, or mascara from under your eyes and, when dampened, can even apply powder eye shadow as eyeliner for an understated look.

• **Magnifying mirror.** Attach a full-size magnifying mirror to your bathroom mirror (mine is 10x) or keep one on a stand nearby. And carry a double-sided compact version in your purse to save yourself from wiggly eyeliner, wandering lipstick, and stray hairs.

• **Your fingers.** Many makeup artists prefer to apply makeup with fingers instead of brushes, especially when using cream formulas, which go on more smoothly when warmed by the heat of your hands. The ring finger in particular gives a light touch and the perfect angle for applying highlighter or blending blush, eyeliner, and concealer, and for dabbing anything under the eyes.

Are You Ready for Your Close-Up?

A lot of us are a bit camera-shy—and we may get even more self-conscious about photo ops as we get older. I've lost count of the number of women who ask me for tips on how to look better in pictures for their professional career, for dating websites, or just to post on Facebook—and I'm happy to share. Because the truth is that with a few tricks, your photos (even selfies!) can keep looking better and better. Here's how to improve your image instantly:

KEEP YOUR CHIN OUT. **When you push your chin slightly out and tilt your head forward, your face and neck look thinner and less jowly.**

FIND YOUR BEST ANGLE. **Most of us have slightly asymmetrical faces, giving us one side that is more photogenic than the other. Go through photos of yourself to see which side is most flattering, then position yourself accordingly at photo time.** *Tip:* **Facing the camera straight on is usually not the best look, but try for yourself.**

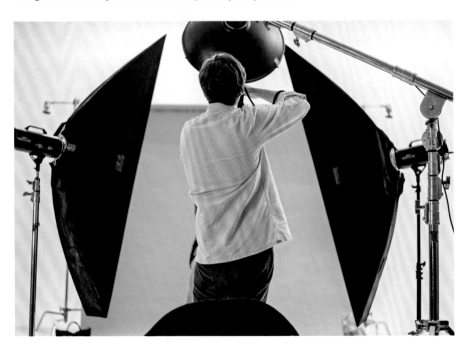

LOOK AT A LIGHT. If there's going to be a flash, focus briefly on a bright light for a few seconds before looking at the camera. This will cause your pupils to constrict, reducing the risk of red-eye.

AVOID OVERHEAD LIGHTS. Lights shining directly above you will cast harsh shadows on your face. Instead, a soft light coming from the side is ideal, especially if it's natural light from a window. *Tip:* **To prevent backlighting, try to face the light rather than having it behind you.**

STAY BELOW THE CAMERA. Looking down at the camera distorts your features and gives most of us extra chins. Instead, make sure the photo is being taken from slightly above your face. That goes for selfies, too.

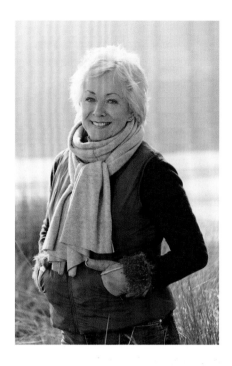

STRIKE A "GLAMOUR POSE." For a great full-length shot, turn your body 45 degrees away from the camera, put your front hand on your hip, shift your weight onto your back leg, pull your back arm a bit behind you, and turn your head to the camera.

DON'T OVERDO THE SMILE. A smile is the best way to look friendly and engaging, but a smile that's too wide or hard can distort your features and look forced. To keep your grin soft and natural, try thinking of something that makes you happy—your spouse, your kids, that tasty dessert you had last night—rather than saying "Cheese."

FOR A BOMBSHELL LOOK, BORROW MARILYN'S "SQUINCH." The "squinch" is a time-tested way of getting a natural and very attractive look in photos—and you don't have to be a screen legend to pull it off. Just narrow your eyes slightly as if you're looking into the distance. Only the lower lids will move, not any other part of your eyes or eyebrows, giving you a flattering look without distorting your features.

GET MAKEUP CAMERA-READY. Dewy skin is great, but a shiny face isn't. Keep some blotting papers in your purse—or use a tissue if you're in a pinch—to pat down your T-zone before the posing starts. If you know photos are on the day's agenda, bump up your brows and your blush to accent your features. And even if it's an impulse photo op, take a second to refresh your lips with a bright pop of color.

the lipstick from feathering. Apply lipstick over the liner, either directly from the tube or using a brush or your finger. Concentrate the lipstick in the center of your mouth, then blend it out to the edges of your lips. Top with a moisturizing balm or light gloss. *Tip:* For a fresh, everyday look, aim for a color just a shade or two darker than your natural tone. Test it by applying it to your lower lip only so you can compare it to your upper lip.

PUT THE PLUMP BACK INTO YOUR POUT
If your lips are looking a little thin, try switching your lip color to fill them back out. Opt for bright peach, pink, and rosy shades with a light shimmer or gloss for maximum pop. Steer clear of overly shiny or glittery formulas, which make skin look dry and dull by comparison. And avoid dark hues, which will make lips look even thinner. *Pro tip:* Instead of adding fullness by tracing dark liner outside your lip line—which looks dated—trace a thin line of highlighter along your upper lip line, then buff it downward with your finger before applying your lip color. The contrast with your lipstick will make lips appear fuller while still looking natural.

Is makeup necessary? Not at all. But smooth skin, defined eyes, and a glow of color on your cheeks and lips can brighten your face and send you out the door ready to take on the world. Keep it up!

Fashion Forward: Great Style Is Habit-Forming

I used to be a dedicated fashionista. Today, I still want to look as chic as possible, but I'm more interested in choosing clothes that don't distract me by riding up, sliding down, pinching, squeezing, or sagging. So instead of tracking trends, I seek out fashion that fits my body and lifestyle, and represents who I am and how I want to show myself to the world. And, really, isn't that what style is all about?

Style Habits for Any Style

The basics of dressing well have nothing to do with age, or fashion sense. By practicing these simple habits, you'll look better every day, whether you're dressing for work, play, or cocktail hour.

> **Stand up straight.** Ann Cuddy wasn't necessarily giving fashion advice, but this habit does double duty. Good posture doesn't just boost your attitude and make you feel more confident; it also makes all your clothes fit better and look more flattering. *Bonus:* It's totally free!

Wear properly fitted underwear. From visible lines to bunched-up briefs, poorly fitting panties can wreck an otherwise impeccable outfit. You don't have to join the thong brigade, but do choose undies that lie flat under your clothes without elastic cutting into your hips or across your butt. If you love a bikini style, try going up a size to get a smoother fit. Or experiment with hipster or boy short panties, which have lower cut legs that disappear better under pants. In any style, look for stretch lace edging, which is softer and less likely to dig than flat elastic. Or choose seamless laser-cut undies from companies like Commando and Hanky Panky, which are designed specifically to avoid panty lines.

Choose uplifting bras. A bra that fits your size and breast shape can reduce back pain, make your clothes fit better, and make you look more shapely (and, yes, younger), too. The right bra should fit smoothly all over, without cutting into your back or shoulders or creating "spillage" out of the top or sides of the cups. Breasts change size and shape over time, so get a professional fitting at least once a year and try a few different styles to see what flatters you the most. But you don't need a huge wardrobe of lingerie (unless you want one!).

- For daily wear, choose two or more everyday bras that offer comfortable support and lift and separate your breasts. Not all bras work with all clothes—or all breasts—so seek bras that suit your shape and complement your favorite necklines. Choose wide-set straps if you love boatneck tops, for instance, or minimizer cups if you wear a lot of button-ups. Alternate them so they each get at least one day off to recover their shape and air out between use, but you don't need to wash them until they're genuinely dirty.

- You also need sports bras with enough support for your favorite activities. Too much bouncing can damage the connective tissue that supports your breasts, leading to sagging. So the larger your breasts and the more high-impact your activities, the more support you'll need. Racerback and T-back styles are especially great, since the straps won't slip when things get sweaty. But make sure they're not too tight! I made the mistake of wearing a tighter-fitting running bra when I competed in a short race recently, and I could barely breathe, because my lungs couldn't expand! And, of course, activewear bras need to stand up to more frequent laundering.

• If you don't want bra straps to show under tanks or strapless dresses, add at least one strapless bra to your lineup, but be sure it fits securely around your rib cage. Styles with silicone or rubber inside the band can help the bra stay put, but they can be irritating if you have sensitive skin. If you're a C cup or bigger, look for wider bands to provide more support and reduce slipping, or try longline styles, which extend to the waist.

• For the most versatility, choose bras that match your skin tone, which will disappear under any color top, especially lighter-hued ones. Add a black option if you wear a lot of dark colors.

• As a rule, bras with underwire provide more lift and separation, but soft-cup or wireless bras are usually more comfortable for weekend or casual wear.

• A contoured foam cup, as in a T-shirt bra, provides a smooth fit under clingy garments and turns down "high beams."

• Hand-wash and air-dry bras to make them last longer.

• Bras stretch over time. When new, the band should fit when you use the outermost hooks. When the band is starting to slip or sag, tighten it up by moving to the next set of hooks. When you're on the last set of hooks, start shopping for a replacement. And adjust the shoulder straps as needed to keep them from slipping. Most bras only last about a year and sports bras lose their supportiveness even sooner.

Smooth out bumps or bulges with shapewear. While industrial-strength girdles mostly disappeared decades ago (thank heaven), contemporary companies like Spanx and Yummie offer a slew of lightly compressive bodysuits, panty hose, shaping shorts, and slips that give you a polished look even under the clingiest dresses. If you want to skip the shapewear, you can still keep your silhouette looking sharp by stocking up on plain tank tops, which make a perfect base layer under cardigans, jackets, blouses, and sweaters. I wear one nearly every day to smooth everything out and to ward off wardrobe malfunctions like gaping button-ups or slipping waistbands. Choose a slim fit that hugs your figure, and be sure it's long enough to stay tucked in. *Tip:* Choose shapewear and base layers that fit closely but comfortably. Sizing down won't make you look thinner; it will just make you miserable.

Shop for fit, not for size. By now we all know that clothing sizes are bogus, right? There are no industry standards, and sizing varies wildly between brands and styles. Instead of fixating on a number when shopping, try on everything that looks like it might fit—regardless of what the label says. And accept that almost no store-bought item is going to be just right. The best plan is to seek styles that flatter your general shape, and buy the size that fits you properly around your biggest part—whether that's hips, shoulders, or bust. Then find a good tailor and have the waist or other parts of the garment taken in.

Dress to flatter the body you have right now. It's tempting to cling to an image of the body you had in your 20s, or the figure you dream of having someday. But if you want to look great right now, you have to dress the body you have today. Six easy ways to do that?

The Art of Letting Go

If your closet is crowded, it's probably time for a purge. Many of us hang on to items that don't fit our bodies or lifestyles, either because we used to love them or because we just want them to work. But the truth is, you'll be happier—and better dressed—if you let them go in favor of clothing that suits the woman you are today. Put another way: We change, so we need our closets to change, too.

Here are two tried-and-true tricks for deciding what to get rid of:

• **The hanger trick.** At the beginning of each season, hang up all your clothes so they face backward. Every time you wear something, turn it around. At the end of the season, anything that hasn't been worn should probably go.

• **Take it all out.** A favorite method of organization experts is to take out every single article of clothing you own and lay it on your bed. Then try on every piece and evaluate it according to how well it fits, how much you like it, and how often you wear it. Put back only the pieces you genuinely love and wear. The rest can go.

Tip: When you do any kind of wardrobe clean-out, try a "time-out" by putting unwanted items in a box or a spare closet for a few weeks. The ones you don't miss can be safely donated or sold without risking purger's remorse.

- **Choose clothing that follows your contours—with some breathing room.** Skin-tight clothes are not only uncomfortable but are unflattering on almost everyone. Conversely, too-baggy clothes add bulk (and years) to your body. For the most flattering line, choose clothes that gently outline your shape and hang just a bit off your body. If you love oversized tops, look for styles with slim-fitting arms to avoid looking dowdy, and pair with fitted bottoms, for balance.

- **Define your waist, no matter how big or small.** Highlight your waist with belts, A-line skirts, wrap dresses and sweaters, and jackets that cinch or nip in at your natural waistline—even if only a little bit. If you're short-waisted, try a skinny belt to keep things in proportion. If you like loose clothing, choose things that either drape to show your form or have just a bit of seaming to hint at your curves. And track down a good tailor, who can add contouring to many "almost perfect" garments.

- **Show a little skin.** Instead of covering yourself from head to toe, be strategic in exposing one body part at a time, which looks both fresh and sophisticated. You don't have to overdo it: Try three-quarter-length sleeves to reveal wrists; V-neck or wide-neck tops to show off your collarbone; or pants cropped just above the ankle. And remember that the most flattering length for a skirt is almost always at the slimmest part of your mid-leg—usually at the knee, or just above or below.

- **Reconsider color.** As with makeup, it's good to reevaluate how your wardrobe colors work with your skin and hair as you get older. Most of us will see our complexion soften over time—making the brightest shades a bit too harsh—and it may take on cooler or warmer undertones that can clash with colors from the opposite camp. If you love bold colors, shift from the most saturated shades to mid-range and jewel tones, which tend to be more flattering. *Tip:* To evaluate the undertone of your skin, look at the veins in your wrist. If they appear blue or purple, you have cool undertones and probably look best in blue, green, or purple. If they look green, you have warm undertones and might want to try red, orange, and yellow shades. And if you see both colors or can't tell, you're probably neutral and can go either way. No matter your undertone, be wary of too much black near your face, where it can make you look washed-out and emphasize dark circles under your eyes. Instead, try less intense neutrals, like charcoal, navy, or chocolate brown. If you must have black, choose a sheer fabric to soften the effect, or add a colorful scarf or bold statement necklace to perk up your complexion.

- **Simplify your silhouette.** Too many ruffles, fringes, bows, and excessive ornamentation can come off as overdone. While there's nothing wrong with being creative, clean lines and bold shapes tend to make you look more elegant and confident than overly fussy outfits. Less really *is* more in fashion, so if you love frills, choose tops and dresses with a draped neckline, ruched waist, or flared peplum rather than a cascade of flounces—and balance them with simple bottoms and accessories.

- **Choose better fabrics.** Yeah, T-shirts are comfy, but cotton jersey isn't flattering in dresses, skirts, or pants, where it can look cheap and clings in all the wrong places. Instead, look for fabrics that drape over your curves and hold their shape when you move, like denser interlock or ponte knits, gabardine, or twill. And while you're at it, upgrade a few of your tees to silk, modal, or linen blends, which hang beautifully and look more polished.

Wardrobe Revamp

Do you need to throw out all your faves just because of the year on your driver's license? No! But don't be afraid to start fresh with a few staples for your current life.

JEANS FOR EVERY BODY

Denim is a wardrobe staple for a reason. But instead of wriggling into those too-tight rhinestone-studded numbers from the juniors department, consider updating your collection with these more flattering styles.

Dark denim mid-rise boot-cut jeans. Ditch the lowriders for a mid-rise fit, which is more comfortable, more flattering, and easier to wear with tops of all lengths. A dark wash without fading or embellishments can be worn almost anywhere, short of a formal event. The wider hem of a boot-cut style looks great with everything from wedges to pumps, and leaves room for booties—a footwear option for almost every occasion. *Tip*: Hem to about a quarter inch off the floor, and make sure the jeans fit comfortably in the butt and hips, with just a little stretch. Take the waist in if necessary.

Dark denim mid-rise straight-leg jeans. Skip the skinnies in favor of a more versatile

> # "Don't go against yourself, don't go against your own nature. It's only going to show."
>
> —DIANE VON FURSTENBERG

straight leg. You can pair them with flats or kitten heels, and tuck them into tall boots in cooler weather. Straight-leg jeans also go beautifully with longer jackets and tunic-length tops.

White boot-cut or straight-leg jeans. As I hope we all know by now, white is a year-round color, and white jeans are a great look anytime. They're perfect for summer with sandals, tanks, or floaty blouses, and always look nautical-chic with a navy jacket. When it gets cooler, pair them with booties, cashmere sweaters, and colorful scarves. *Tip:* For an invisible look under any white pant, choose underwear in a shade that matches your skin tone, rather than white, which will stand out.

DON'T GIVE UP THE DRESSES
Dresses make almost everyone feel pretty and are easy to throw on in a flash. But leave the baby-dolls and flounced sleeves for the preschool set. Instead, opt for these three time-tested styles that work beautifully on grown-up women:

Wrap dresses with long or three-quarter-length sleeves look great on almost everyone. Tie the belt on the side to avoid emphasizing your middle—and use a simple knot rather than a bow for a more sophisticated look. Add pumps or boots and you're dressed.

Sleeveless sheath dresses that skim your shape can be worn alone or with fitted cardigans or jackets, making them adaptable for almost any occasion. You can also change the whole look of a sleeveless dress by layering it over a slim fitting turtleneck or crewneck bodysuit for cooler weather.

"Fit and flare" dresses are fitted on top, and flare out below the waist, creating a swingy look that accentuates your waist and balances most figures. Great for dancing, too!

If you have at least one perfectly fitting dress in any of these styles, you'll have an instant outfit to dress up or down as needed.

CONSIDER THE COMPLETERS

If most of your wardrobe is composed of separates, like slacks, skirts, and simple tops, completers are a great way to pull a look together and show off your style.

Fitted cardigans can turn anything into a finished outfit and can be worn open to show off other layers. Both long and three-quarter sleeves work well. To wear with skirts and dresses, look for cuts that end just at or above the hip. Longer cardigans are great with straight-leg jeans or pants.

Structured jackets can be worn as outerwear or layered over lightweight tanks and tees for a polished everyday ensemble. And there's something for every style—from edgy asymmetrical or moto looks to practical cargo styles to trim wool blazers or go-with-anything jean jackets. For the most flattering lines, choose jackets that fit smoothly in the shoulders and have trim sleeves and contoured waists. Cropped jackets that end just at or above the waist are especially great with dresses.

Scarves are ideal for adding color and pattern to an outfit as well as helping you adapt to unpredictable weather—or your own personal heat waves. They can provide some cover if you're self-conscious about showing too much skin, and can reduce the contrast between your face and clothing colors that would otherwise overwhelm you. Floaty silk scarves can be knotted or draped around your neck. Casual cotton options add drape and sun protection to summer outfits. And cashmere, pashmina, or wool scarves wrapped lightly around your neck can turn a plain sweater-and-slacks combo into a great winter look, especially paired with boots.

Shoes are almost everybody's favorite accessory. And for good reason! Shoes set the tone for your entire look, from polished patent pumps to slouchy suede booties. But comfortable shoes make a huge difference to your health and happiness. Poorly fitted shoes will cause foot and back pain and discourage you from walking—and we want to walk more, not less. Trendy is fine, but look for styles with a sturdy sole, adequate cushioning, and a toe box big enough to avoid squeezing your piggies. If you love pointy-toe shoes, find a pair where the point starts past your toes to avoid discomfort. If you love higher heels, wedges with a little platform under the front will give you height and arch support. Or, for walkable everyday glamour, ballet flats, cool oxfords, or kitten heels look great. My favorite shoe trend is the box heel, which combines comfort and stability. For more formal occasions, try a sculpted heel around two to three inches high. Leopard or snake print adds a touch of the exotic to any outfit. And if you want to buy only one fab pair of evening shoes, look for bronze or pewter, because these colors go with everything.

Over the years, I've learned that looking good isn't about pleasing other people; it's about building my own confidence. If you feel good, you look good. If you look good, you're confident. If you're confident ... there's nothing you can't do.

10 Small Steps to Always Looking the Part

❶ Stand up straight and tall.

❷ Shampoo less, condition more.

❸ Choose a style (and a stylist) that works with your hair, not against it.

❹ Review makeup and clothing colors every couple of years to assess how they work with your skin and hair.

❺ Keep makeup light and bright.

❻ Add magnifying mirrors to your bathroom and purse—and use them.

❼ Dress the body you have today.

❽ Only wear clothes that fit.

❾ Replace bras once a year.

❿ Let go of anything that doesn't suit the woman you are now.

Dressing for Your Best Self

The most flattering look? Good health and a confident smile. But most of us feel even more fab when we also know that our clothes are accentuating our positives (and glossing over the negatives). If that's you, consider these tried-and-true wardrobe tricks.

INSTEAD OF HIDING YOUR BEST FEATURES,

Play them up by wearing a mix of darker colors and light colors. Get strategic! Wear lighter and brighter shades on the parts of your body you want to show off, and darker colors on the parts you'd like to downplay. If you feel bottom-heavy and want balance, draw more attention to your upper half by pairing simple dark pants or a skirt with an attention-grabbing top and bold earrings. If your weight distribution is reversed, change the emphasis: Wear a simple dark top with a gorgeous print skirt or bold slacks.

INSTEAD OF MIXING CLOTHES AND ACCESSORIES THAT CUT YOUR BODY IN HALF,

Choose items and colors that make you look longer and leaner. Stick to one color from head to toe—or use accent colors in vertical lines on pieces like long cardigans, vests, or color-blocked dresses. Try to avoid breaking up your body with horizontal lines, wide belts, or waistbands. For the longest-looking legs, skip the ankle straps and expose as much of the foot as possible—or match your pants or tights to your shoes.

INSTEAD OF BEING SELF-CONSCIOUS ABOUT OUT-OF-SHAPE ARMS,

Camouflage with flair. Pair sleeveless shirts and dresses with a lightweight jacket or open-front cardigan. In warm weather, add a little coverage with a sheer blouse layered over a cami. And try poet-style tops with billowy sleeves and "cold shoulder" tops—but balance them with more fitted pants to avoid looking bigger all over.

INSTEAD OF FEELING OVEREXPOSED BY SKIMPY SUMMER DRESSES,

Try a maxi or midi. A maxi or midi dress can keep you chic and covered at the same time. If you're short, skip full-skirted options in favor of a sleeker fit that makes you look like a long column. And look for cool, floaty dresses in comfortable fabrics that hit the most flattering part of your leg: the knee. Add a wedge shoe for extra height and style.

INSTEAD OF FOCUSING ONLY ON WHAT'S HAPPENING BELOW THE NECK,

Wear clothes that flatter your face. Wearing lighter, brighter colors around your face will draw attention upward and will add luminosity to help you look more vibrant and awake.

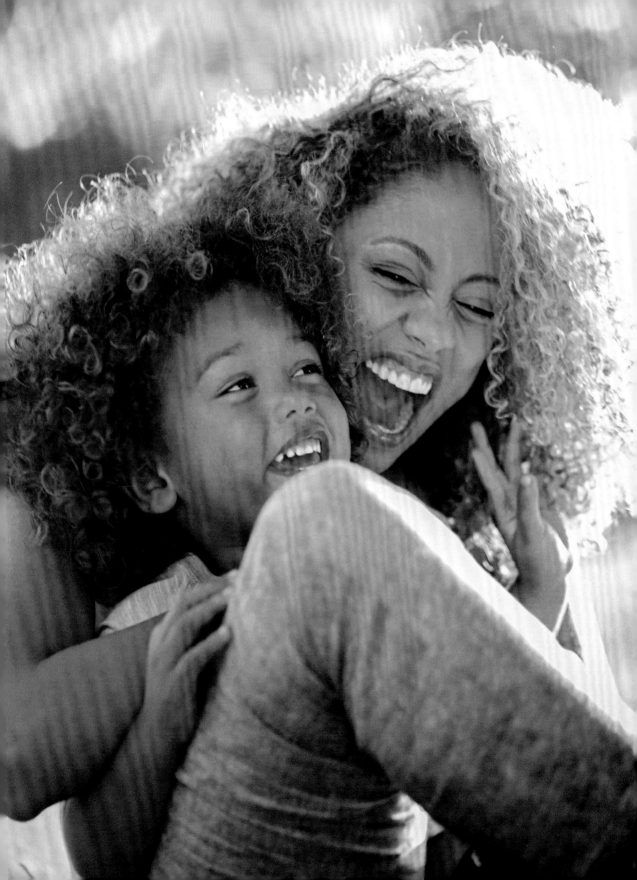

CHAPTER 12

Happiness Matters

"Optimism is the faith that leads to achievement;
nothing can be done without hope or confidence."

—HELEN KELLER

A friend once told me that when she thinks of me, she pictures a glass half full, never half empty. She said she appreciated my natural tendency to be optimistic, always looking for the positive.

That made me happy.

Well, "it" didn't actually make me happy, because according to a lot of research, only "I" can make myself happy. Sure, compliments and good experiences can enhance our enjoyment of life—temporarily. And negative experiences can definitely darken our day. But the power is within each of us to find our own happy place, even if you're naturally a "glass half empty" sort of person.

And it's worth finding that place, because a sunny-side-up attitude might help you live a better—and possibly longer—life. Science says, "Cheer up."

- A 2015 study that evaluated data from more than 30,000 Americans found a strong correlation between reported happiness and a longer life, which was consistent regardless of other circumstances, like health, education level, marital status, or financial situation.

- Researchers from University College London measured the happiness of 3,800 people between the ages of 52 and 79 and then tracked their health. After five

> **"I am still determined to be cheerful and happy, in whatever situation I may be; for I have also learned…that the greater part of our happiness or misery depends upon our dispositions."**
>
> —MARTHA WASHINGTON

years, 7 percent of the least happy people had died, compared to 4 percent of the happiest people. The researchers then estimated that happy older people are 35 percent less likely to die within five years than unhappy folks—even after all other factors are taken into consideration.

• The "Nun Study"—an ongoing project started in 1986 and conducted by the University of Kentucky—has tracked several hundred nuns over the course of decades. Data includes autobiographical essays the sisters wrote when they entered the convent as young women. Of the nuns who have died since the study began, those who wrote the most positive essays in their youth lived an average of 10 years longer than those with the most negative outlooks. Even more intriguingly, the happiest nuns were least likely to develop dementia or Alzheimer's—and if they did develop it, they showed fewer symptoms, suggesting that happier brains may have a built-in defense system.

• A study from the Harvard School of Public Health reported that optimists are less likely to develop heart disease and cardiovascular problems than pessimists.

BUT HOW DOES OUR MOOD AFFECT OUR WELL-BEING?
The relationship between happiness and health is multifaceted, and not all of it is

LOVE YOUR AGE

clearly understood. One known aspect is that as happiness goes up, stress goes down. And since stress suppresses the immune system and contributes to heart disease and other chronic illnesses, anything that reduces it will probably help us live longer and better. But there may be some other benefits to a good attitude as well.

- A Carnegie Mellon University study found that people who demonstrate positive emotions are less likely to become ill after being exposed to a cold virus.

- People who maintain a positive outlook and engage in positive behaviors don't produce as much cortisol, the stress hormone. In excess doses, cortisol can raise blood pressure, reduce bone density, suppress thyroid function, interfere with blood sugar regulation, and disrupt sleep.

- People who regularly suppress their emotions tend to have higher blood pressure, as well as a higher risk of heart disease and cancer than people who express their feelings—both good and bad.

It's No Joke—Laughing Improves Your Life

- Physicians at the University of Maryland discovered that hearty laughter immediately expands blood vessels and increases blood flow almost as much as aerobic exercise.

- Laughter improves memory by almost 45 percent, which may be why funny advertisements tend to be 25 percent more effective than other ads.

- Both men and women are more attracted to partners who laugh.

- Managers with a good sense of humor are perceived as better leaders.

- Women laugh more than men do, but men and women both tend to laugh more at men. (Ha!)

- Laughter is contagious. Social laughter occurs 30 times more often than solitary laughter.

- Laughing out loud boosts immune activity, can reduce pain and stress, and enhances sleep.

- Laughter also activates the endorphin system, which can further increase feelings of optimism and happiness.

On top of all that, happiness has been proved to elevate our mood, improve our sleep, make us more attractive to potential mates (this is true for both genders), propel us forward with our goals, improve our ability to resolve conflicts, and create stronger relationships. Oh, and it feels great, too.

Programmed for the Sunny Side of the Street

I'll admit it, a Pollyanna attitude comes a little easier to me than to some others. I've definitely had my ups and downs in life, but I've always felt that I was predisposed to be cheerful. And that turns out to be true! Several recent studies involving identical twins, including one from the University of Minnesota, have established that as much as 50 percent of our ability to be happy is actually programmed into our genetic makeup.

However, even if finding the positive is more difficult for you, I have some very happy news: You can change.

Expect Less, Get More

A study published in 2015 in the *Journal of Experimental Psychology* revealed that when we try too hard to make ourselves happy, we often end up less so. The theory is that if we're aspiring to a certain kind of experience—like a dream vacation or a storybook wedding—we can easily become frustrated if things don't work out exactly as we planned, leaving us unable to appreciate the good things that happened instead. (Americans in particular struggle with this, because we tend to focus so much on our individual happiness and material success that we overlook the value of our relationships and social experiences, which provide an emotional buffer in more community-minded cultures.)

Neuroscientists at University College London arrived at a similar conclusion by using an MRI machine that evaluated volunteers' brains while they played a game. The scientists then adapted the game for smartphones and recruited 18,000 additional players to test their findings. In both settings, winning or losing didn't affect happiness nearly as much as whether the final score was better or worse than the players had anticipated.

The British team even developed an equation that was able to accurately predict how happy people would feel while playing their game—essentially creating mathematical proof that the secret to happiness really *is* having low expectations.

Think of happiness like body temperature; we each have a genetically influenced set point, but our environment and behaviors can change our actual experience. DNA can get us halfway there ... but the rest is up to us.

What's the Secret to Happiness?

That's the big question, right? What makes us happy?

Well, we know it's not money. Way back in the 1970s, psychologist Philip Brickman published a famous study revealing that people who had won the lottery were no happier than those who hadn't. And in 2010 a team of researchers, including Nobel laureate Daniel Kahneman, published an analysis of 450,000 people that confirmed that as long as we can afford the basic necessities of life, happiness doesn't rise proportionately with cash flow.

And success doesn't make us happy, either. In fact, psychologist and happiness guru Shawn Achor argues it's the other way around: The happier we are, the more successful we are. As he explains in his book *The Happiness Advantage,* our brains work better when we're feeling positive, so developing a sunny disposition will result in making us smarter, more creative, and more successful. Other research confirms his assertion, finding that optimists tend to get better jobs and more promotions, and have more success in athletic endeavors.

What, then, is the key to total, complete 100 percent happiness? Other than, as Charlie Brown would say, a warm puppy? (Although, speaking from experience, I can tell you a warm puppy can help.)

Some psychologists and social scientists who study happiness define it as a subjective sense of well-being that includes:

- Self-acceptance

- Personal growth and pursuit of goals

- Positive social relationships

- Autonomy

- A sense of control over your own life

Happiness isn't nonstop giddiness; it's a deep and comforting sense of contentment that persists in spite of life's challenges and setbacks. In general, people who describe themselves as happy tend not to worry too much (especially about things they can't control), they accept their own personal shortcomings, they're conscientious, and they have strong social connections.

That means for most of us, these are the biggest factors influencing our ability—or inability—to enjoy life:

• Meaningful relationships with family, friends, a spouse, a faith community, or other groups (even just having a pet can contribute greatly to happiness)

• Pleasurable experiences, like enjoying a sunset, concert, or good meal on a regular basis

• A sense of accomplishment, whether from finishing a painting or starting a business

• Feeling that life has meaning, which might come from religion, philosophy, or purposeful work

• Good health (because without it, it's pretty hard to enjoy everything else)

Bad Stress vs. Good Stress

Stress isn't all bad. Occasional bouts deliver a burst of adrenaline and other hormones that sharpen your senses, spurring you to action when you need to finish a work deadline or if you encounter a ferocious animal (human or otherwise) and need to make a run for it. That's "good stress."

But when the same hormones are released in a steady stream for weeks, months, or years, it's "bad stress," which can keep your heart rate too high while suppressing your immune system. Low-grade but chronic stress—due to financial troubles, an unhappy relationship, or a demanding job, for example—can lead to severe biological changes that can slowly poison your body, contributing to heart disease, high blood pressure, severe inflammation, and even asthma.

Don't let chronic stress rule your life. Identify the source of your stress and take action to eliminate or at least minimize it. And use the tips in this chapter to start building your own happiness habits.

In addition, studies show we are happiest when we are living in the moment and our minds are focused on the present, not the past or future. That's why exercises like mindfulness meditation put most people in a positive mood. Sounds good to me!

Want to Be Happy? Start by Being Grateful

Gratitude helps you focus on what you *do* have instead of what you don't—and research has confirmed that it's an essential ingredient to happiness. Appreciation increases your sense of peace and contentment, allows you to better accept your own strengths and weaknesses, and helps you feel closer to people and things outside yourself.

Being grateful:

- Helps you sleep better

- Makes you more likely to exercise

- Strengthens your immune system

- Reduces stress

- Increases your sense of belonging

- Makes you more likely to remember positive things

- Rewrites negative or neutral memories to be more positive

- Increases productivity

Studies conducted by positive psychology pioneer Martin Seligman showed that when people sent or read letters of gratitude to others who had not been properly thanked for past kindnesses, most letter writers experienced a huge increase in happiness and a dramatic drop in depression. Try it! You'll find you can reach the same levels of happiness even if you write a gratitude letter that you can't send (for example, to someone who has passed away).

Simply taking a few moments during the day to think about the things for which you are grateful can give you real benefits, whether you do that by journaling, by silently "counting your blessings," or through prayer.

Filling the Empty Nest

For many parents, the moment when grown kids finally move out can trigger an emotional upheaval. When both my daughters left for college at the same time (one of them to Scotland!), it really created a vacuum in our home. I missed the noise and the chaotic feel of having four people under the same roof, even though sometimes it's nice to have a little peace and quiet for a change. So I can testify that the so-called empty-nest syndrome is incredibly real. It's also very common among both men and women, and can lead to serious depression if it isn't acknowledged and addressed. And no wonder! We've spent at least 18 years building our identity around parenthood and now that identity is being rocked. If it feels like you don't know who you are anymore, that may be because you don't!

So how can you embrace the next phase of your life with joy?

ACCEPT IT. Remind yourself—hourly if needed—that this is a natural part of having kids. It's normal to feel grief (although not everyone does), so treat this loss with as much compassion as you would with any other—then move through it. It might take time for you to adjust to your new role, but clinging to the past isn't an answer.

ACKNOWLEDGE IT. No doubt about it, your relationship with your children is going to evolve now that they're adults. Simply talking about this new reality can help—especially if they're going to be coming home when they're on break from college or the military. Ask what they want from you now, discuss what you're willing to do for them, and be open about what you expect in return. Whatever the issue, address it as if you're both adults—because you are.

RESIST THE TEMPTATION TO MANAGE YOUR CHILD'S LIFE. You've had almost two decades to teach them how to cope with the world. It's time to step back and let them live their lives, which includes making mistakes. Yes, it's hard, but trying to control an adult child is unhealthy for both of you. Take it from me, a professional nagger: Dole out advice only when asked ... and then let it go.

GET TO KNOW THE PERSON YOUR CHILD IS BECOMING. You know who has great relationships with their grown children? The parents who don't keep trying to see their kids as they were when they were little but who accept them for who they are today. And this will help you, too, because it will keep you grounded in the new reality rather than constantly revisiting memories of kindergarten.

FOCUS ON YOURSELF. You might need a little time to remember who you are and what you love to do, but chances are good you enjoy something beyond just parenting, so either rekindle a dormant interest or find a new one. Parenthood doesn't define you; it's just one part of the rich tapestry of your life. This might be the perfect time to start traveling a bit, spend more time with people you haven't seen for a while, or even start a new career. The world will open up its many possibilities and opportunities if you let it. *Tip:* If your kids are still at home, start cultivating your own interests now so the transition won't feel so abrupt.

CHANNEL THAT ENERGY. Look at all the other parts of your identity, including roles like wife, daughter, business owner or employee, community member, friend, athlete, artist, etc. Can you put more time and effort into one of these roles now that your "Mom" job is less demanding? If not, can you create an entirely new role for yourself?

And if you're married, here's some extra good news: A study from Harvard recently found that marital satisfaction tends to increase around the same time those sweet but pesky kids leave home. Coincidence?

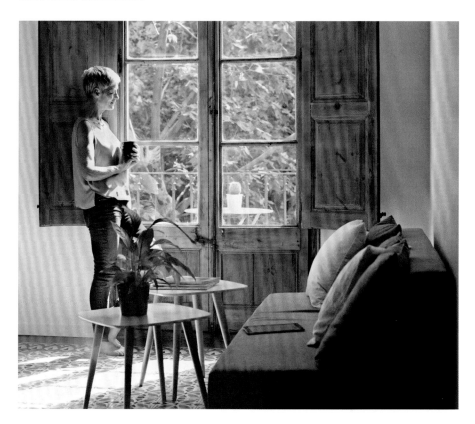

Let's Take This Outside

Another reliable way to bring more contentment into your life—and get a near-instant mood lift—is as simple as opening your door. Just a few minutes outdoors can lower stress, raise your energy, and improve your happiness.

• According to a study from the University of Rochester, stepping outside boosts energy levels for 90 percent of people. Another study from the same team found that spending time in nature leads people to value community and relationships more and to be more generous with money.

• Japanese researchers have found that spending time in forested settings reduces stress markers like blood pressure, heart rate, and cortisone production, and boosts the part of the nervous system responsible for relaxation. Other studies have found that just looking at pictures of nature can lower physical stress responses.

• A 2010 study at Britain's University of Essex concluded that as little as five minutes a day of any activity conducted in a "green" or "natural" setting produces measurable benefits in mental and physical health.

• Stanford researchers found that a 90-minute walk in a natural environment reduces stress, depression, and negative rumination even more effectively than a similar walk in an urban environment. A separate study conducted by researchers in the United Kingdom found that group nature walks are an effective method for improving mood and helping people cope with stress, especially during a loss or life transition.

• Hospital patients with window views of trees may heal faster and need less pain medication than patients with views of a brick wall.

• Research from Washington State University has found that just adding a few houseplants to your space can reduce stress and mental fatigue.

So it seems our mothers were right when they said a little fresh air would do us good. And it's not hard to find! Put a few plants in your living room; take a walk to the park on the corner; or drink a cup of tea out on your balcony. There—don't you feel better?

Give Your Brain a Break Today

Got that overflowing-calendar buzzing-brain syndrome? One of the serious side effects of living a go-go life all the time is that we increase our

Caring for Caregivers

According to AARP, an estimated 43.5 million adults reported providing care for another person, and 60 percent of these caregivers are women, with an average age of 49. Caregiving can be gratifying and meaningful, but it can also be physically and emotionally challenging. While caregivers face some unique challenges, the basic strategies for reducing stress still apply:

• **Take care of you.** You can't help your loved one if you're burned out. Eat well every day, and treat any medical issues of your own promptly.

• **Get enough sleep and rest.** Find ways, even if you have to hire overnight help.

• **Get adequate exercise.** Moving your body will not only reduce stress but will benefit your overall health and increase your energy for dealing with caregiving.

• **Prioritize and delegate.** Martyrdom is not the path to happiness. Instead of trying to do it all, make a list of what needs to be done, and seek assistance wherever possible, including from medical professionals, local nonprofits, community service agencies, and other relatives. And don't be afraid to ask your employer for a more flexible schedule during this time.

• **Take breaks.** Recruit other family members, look into adult day care, or hire help, but find a way to arrange time for yourself at least a couple of times every week.

• **Let your emotions out.** Caregiving can be emotionally overwhelming, combining fear and anxiety with frustration and anger. If you have a supportive friend willing to let you vent, then don't be shy. Otherwise, look for a therapist, support group, or online forum to help you process your feelings.

• **Stay social.** Caregiving can be very isolating for both you and your loved one, so it's important to prioritize relationships with other people, whether that means inviting extended family over for potluck dinners or setting up a standing date to exercise or visit a museum with a friend.

• **Be present in the moment.** Ruminating on how you wish things were different or worrying about whether you're doing something right will only increase stress and depression. Instead, give your full attention to whatever task you're doing—whether it's work, caregiving, or taking a restorative hike. And take a few minutes to simply sit and breathe calmly.

For help and resources, visit AARP's Caregiving Resource Center at *aarp.org/caregiving*.

stress levels far beyond what our bodies and brains can handle, making ourselves tense and irritable in the short term—and increasing our risk of illnesses in the long term. When we're strung out, we feel like we're working hard, but most of us aren't as creative or effective as we could otherwise be, which means we end up even more stressed, creating a vicious cycle of busyness that always keeps us running behind. Not fun!

But the great news is that you can break that cycle and counteract that stress with the simple time-tested strategy of meditation. It sounds too good to be true, I know, but giving your tense, distracted brain a rest—by spending a few minutes focused on something as simple as your breath—can turn your whole day around.

What's more, many studies indicate that meditation can actually change the physical structure of your brain, creating more positive emotions and leading to greater happiness and well-being. An increasing number of mental health professionals are now using mindfulness meditation in conjunction with other therapies to help reduce negative, self-defeating thoughts and even to effectively treat depression and anxiety.

Ode to Joy

There's no question about it: Music improves overall health and well-being, and lifts our spirits. Want to harness that power? Choose the right music for the moment. If you want to relax and let your emotions out, think classical (Beethoven—my all-time favorite—can bring me to tears anytime). If you want to energize your workout, turn up fast-paced rock or dance music. If you're feeling lonely, choose lyrics that give you a sense of connection. No matter what you pick, try adding some music to every day.

And to get the most out of your melodies, sing along. Engaging actively with music releases endorphins and strengthens the immune system even more than just passively listening. Sing in the shower, sing along with the radio, or grab a mike at karaoke night. For the biggest happiness boost of all, join a choir! Choir members experience benefits including stronger social networks, reduced depression, and even improved posture.

MEDITATION FOR LIFE
Mindfulness meditation is a powerful technique taught in many cultures, but it's easy to do on your own. To start, sit comfortably in a chair or cross-legged on the floor. Close your eyes and focus only on your breathing. Breathe in deeply and slowly through your nose, filling your belly, not just your chest. Breathe out slowly. You will probably have some thoughts coming into your head, so notice them but try not to

get caught up in them. Just let them drift by like clouds. Whenever you notice that you're getting distracted by a thought, gently refocus your attention on your breathing. That's it—you're meditating!

Start with five minutes a day, and if you enjoy it, try extending your meditation gradually to 30 minutes or more. There are many other ways to practice meditation, including while walking or running. You can even try an app like Insight Timer to help guide you in and out of your sessions. If you meditate regularly, it will help you realize that you're in control of your thoughts and emotions and will help you maintain perspective about things going on around you. And that, as you might expect, can make you happier.

The Ups and Downs of Our Emotional Lives

For most of us, every day brings a range of feelings, which all add richness and depth to our life experience. And, while most of us prefer joy to sadness, negative emotions are important for helping us process what we're going through. (This might explain why, of the 2,000 English words that describe emotions, only 30 percent are for positive feelings.)

The older we get, the more likely we are to face events that can increase feelings like anxiety, grief, and anger. From the distress over an empty nest, a health scare, or a career change, to the agony caused by divorce or the loss of our own parents, adulthood brings a host of challenging emotions. How do we navigate them without giving in to pessimism?

> **Don't fight the feelings.** True happiness is about weathering the storms of life with equanimity, not staying stuck on your "smile" setting at all times. Grief, in particular, often comes in waves of despair that might be broken up with moments of peace and even laughter. Allow yourself to be comfortable with whatever feeling is happening right now. If you must put on a cheerful face, give yourself permission to have a good cry afterward. And if you find yourself becoming emotional at an inopportune time, just excuse yourself and trust others to understand. Don't waste time on embarrassment.
>
> **Accept reality.** Almost nothing increases unhappiness as quickly as dwelling on woulda-coulda-shouldas. You don't have to like the situation you're in, but don't make it worse by pretending it isn't happening. Mindfulness

Quick Ways to Boost Your Happiness

In just a few minutes, you can improve your mood—and your life—by adding some positive practices to your daily routine. And they don't cost a thing.

WRITE. Especially if you're feeling irritable or unhappy, journaling for a few minutes can reduce stress and increase positive feelings. Try to focus on things for which you feel grateful or things that are going well for you.

MEDITATE. Even a short meditation can reduce your heart rate and cortisol production, and may protect against depression and anxiety.

CALL. Phone a friend or relative just to chat. Women with strong social networks deal with stress better, have higher self-esteem, lower risk of memory disorders, and lower blood pressure, and may even live longer.

LISTEN. Pay attention when someone is talking to you. Empathetic listening can boost general well-being as well as social connectedness.

DANCE. It's great for your body and your physical fitness, of course, but dance affects your mind much like meditation, resulting in an increase in relaxation, confidence, and healthy processing of emotion.

WALK. Take a walk outside. Regular exercise and connectedness to nature are both linked to a positive attitude.

NAP. If you feel like your day needs a reset, take a 20-minute nap. Not only does lack of sleep inhibit optimism, but shutting off your mind for a while might help you shift perspective. Keep it short, though, or you could end up more groggy than refreshed.

CHECK IT OFF. Checking items off a to-do list can make you feel more satisfied with your day. Or write a "things I've done" list, which has been shown to be just as effective and often more cheering.

and therapy—particularly cognitive behavioral therapy—can help with acceptance, but so can just writing down the bare facts of a situation and reading them aloud until you believe them.

Be open to the moment. Every phase of life offers its own particular benefits and challenges. If you fixate on what used to be, you cut yourself off from what you have now and what might be coming next. One trick of experienced mindfulness practitioners is to avoid labeling circumstances as "good" or "bad" and instead to simply describe them in neutral terms. This also helps avoid clinging to negative emotions for too long. Instead of fixating on how angry you are, for instance, try saying: "I'm feeling really angry right now." It seems like a trivial difference, but learning to distinguish between your permanent self and your temporary feelings is incredibly powerful. Feelings come and go, but your true self remains.

Find strength in numbers. We all think we're special, but no matter how painful the experience you're having, the odds are better than good that other people have already been through something similar. Tapping into their collective wisdom will reduce feelings of isolation and loneliness, and can give you great strategies for coping, too. Find a support group or counselor specializing in your issue or seek out memoirs and movies about people in similar situations.

10 Surefire Ways to ...

GET UNHAPPY	GET HAPPY
❶ Wallow in negative thoughts.	❶ Count your blessings.
❷ Be judgmental of yourself and others.	❷ Practice compassion—for everyone.
❸ Hold onto grudges.	❸ Forgive and move on.
❹ Isolate yourself.	❹ Stay engaged with life.
❺ Overcommit yourself.	❺ Be mindful of how you spend your time.
❻ Spend too much time on social media.	❻ Cultivate relationships that nourish you.
❼ Procrastinate.	❼ Get information, then act.
❽ Put yourself last.	❽ Prioritize your own well-being.
❾ Compare yourself to others.	❾ Accept yourself as you are.
❿ Leave depression and anxiety untreated.	❿ Take good care of your mental and physical health.

Use all the tools at your disposal. By now, you know that exercise, sleep, social contact, laughter, music, healthy food, mindfulness, gratitude, and exposure to nature can all help to stabilize your mood. You may have your own time-tested mental health boosters, too. So use them all. Will a long walk in the woods or a night at the ballet erase a difficult situation? No, but taking good care of yourself physically and mentally can help you feel more at peace and will reduce the chance that unpleasant experiences will trigger serious depression or other stress-related health issues.

Down for a Day ... or Depressed?

One of the key things to remember about happiness is that it's a long-term measure of our emotional well-being, not a minute-by-minute assessment. If we feel generally content with our lives, then that feeling persists even when our mood is sad or angry—or at least it returns quickly after a good cry or a cathartic run. So if you're having a rough day (or week), just hang in there. Even the sunniest among us have moments when we want to pull a blanket over our heads.

But if this feeling continues for more than a couple of weeks, it could indicate depression, which can be triggered by changes in brain chemistry, hormonal imbalances, underlying health issues, social isolation, external events—or a combination of factors. Depression isn't just a lack of happiness; it's a serious medical condition that can cause a domino effect of mental and physical ailments if not treated promptly.

Women suffering from depression don't just cry a lot—although that is a common symptom—but they often have a loop of negative thoughts running through their head over and over, beating them down with guilt, self-criticism, and hopelessness. They may feel physically exhausted and mentally foggy—as if their brain is shutting down. They may have dramatic reactions to seemingly trivial things, and often feel that they cannot control their emotions. Left untreated, depression can drag down our immune system, damage our cardiovascular health, and cause other diseases, too.

What's more, many people don't realize how common depression is, especially as we age.

• Sixteen million Americans over 18 suffer from depression each year, and women are almost twice as likely to experience a depressive episode as men.

• Depression frequently occurs in tandem with anxiety—and the two conditions can exacerbate each other.

• Nearly 24 percent of women over 64 take an antidepressant, and 11 percent of women between 45 and 64 take antianxiety medications.

• Older patients suffering from depression have 50 percent higher overall health care costs than older patients who don't have depression.

Clearly, depression can have a dramatic impact on your health and quality of life. And, if you've been depressed for a while, it might be hard to imagine feeling good again. But depression usually responds very well to treatment, which might involve counseling, mindfulness practice, medication, or a combination. So call your doctor if you:

• Have been experiencing long, deep feelings of sadness

• Have started sleeping more or less than usual

• Have been feeling emotionally numb

• Have trouble making decisions

• Struggle with focusing your mind or completing tasks

• Feel guilty or worthless

• Have a loss of interest in things that used to interest you, including sex

• Have started eating more or less than usual

• Have had unexplained weight loss or gain

• Find yourself thinking about death or how you might kill yourself

As scary as depression is, it is also very common and, for some, very treatable. So if you think you're depressed, don't wait. Things can get better if you get help.

How Not to Undermine Your Own Happiness

One of the amazing things about being human is that we have a huge amount of control over how we experience our lives. But instead of using that power to promote peace and contentment, many of us undermine our happiness by making the same unhelpful choices again and again. These bad mental habits can be just as unhealthy—and just as addicting—as junk food habits, and they clog up our brains the same way that french fries clog our arteries. So if you catch yourself sliding toward the dark side, try to implement a strategy for happiness instead.

Why Talking to Yourself Is Anything but Crazy

I'm a big believer in talking to myself. In fact, I've made "me" my #1 closest advisor. And I'm not crazy! Lots of experts think self-talk can be a powerful ally for your happiness and health. But if the voices in your head are negative, they can actually decrease your capacity for happiness, undermine your best instincts, and create a cascade of mental and physical problems. Instead, learn how to harness the power of self-talk for good.

• **Pay attention to any negative statements you say to yourself,** especially if you repeat them over and over. Things like "I'm so disorganized" or "I can't do anything right" can become so ingrained in your subconscious that you don't even realize you're saying them.

• **Identify where and when these statements originated.** Whether it's something that was said to you, or something you first said to yourself as a reaction to a painful experience, finding the source of negative self-talk can help you stop it.

• **Realize that these statements aren't helping you move forward.** Some criticisms may have once had some basis in reality, but many are totally false.

Either way, continually rehashing them doesn't allow you to enjoy your life as it is today, so let them all go. If you can, forgive the person who first said them. And forgive yourself for believing them.

• **Be proactive.** "Confirmation bias" describes the brain's tendency to seek out evidence to support the beliefs it already holds. You can use that bias to your advantage by replacing any negative self-talk with positive statements (even if you don't quite believe them yet!). If you repeatedly tell your brain, "I'm confident and competent," for example, it will be more likely to notice events that demonstrate your best qualities.

• **Repeat your affirmations daily.** Say them out loud at least every morning and night, and repeat them in your head while waiting in line, exercising, or driving. Chances are the old negative phrases have been repeating themselves while you were doing these activities, so it's time to take charge and replace them with positive thoughts.

Bottom line? The way you talk to yourself actually matters, so choose your words carefully.

Best Foods for a Better Mood

No surprise here! What you eat affects your mood the same way it affects everything else. And, also no surprise, what's good for your heart and brain is also good for your happiness. Many studies have found that a diet rich in fish, olive oil, nuts, and lots of plant-based foods is linked to lower rates of depression and higher levels of happiness. You'll get particularly blissful benefits from:

Dark leafy greens. Kale, collard greens, spinach, bok choy, and other greens are rich in folate, magnesium, and other nutrients that help regulate brain chemistry to keep your mood more balanced.

Dark chocolate. It's true! The antioxidants found in cocoa beans can calm us down and make us feel more content. Look for dark chocolate with at least 70 percent cacao.

Fatty fish. Salmon, catfish, herring, tuna, sardines, and other fatty fish offer an abundance of omega-3 fatty acids, which support brain chemicals linked with mood, including dopamine and serotonin. If fish isn't your fave, consider fish oil capsules or find an omega-3 supplement made from algae. The exact dose may vary, so talk to your doctor or try starting with one gram (1,000 milligrams) daily and aim for a formula that contains roughly twice as much EPA as DHA.

Shellfish. A deficiency in vitamin B_{12} may contribute to depression and anxiety, but shellfish such as mussels, oysters, and clams all contain high levels of this important nutrient. Vegetarian-friendly B_{12} supplements of up to 100 micrograms daily work well, too.

Saffron. This spice works almost like Prozac to treat depression, according to some studies. It appears to help regulate the neurotransmitters in the brain and may even boost levels of the feel-good chemical serotonin, putting them into high gear. Sprinkle it into rice to add an exotic uplift to your pilafs.

Legumes. Beans—especially chickpeas, lentils, and black-eyed peas—are loaded with folate and zinc, two nutrients that are particularly effective against depression.

Probiotics. There is a proven link between our mood and the bacteria levels in our gut. Fermented foods, such as sauerkraut and kimchi, contain big doses of the beneficial bacteria known as probiotics, which have been shown to alleviate depression and social anxiety. Probiotics are also available in supplement form. There are many different ways to get your daily dose of probiotics, including capsules and gummies, so talk with your doctor or nutritionist to determine the best option for you.

Nuts and seeds. Vitamin E contributes to a better mood, and nuts such as almonds, hazelnuts, and walnuts are terrific sources. Chia seeds and pumpkin seeds, in turn, are good sources of magnesium, zinc, and certain omega-3s.

Choose Happiness

Happiness should not be a goal in and of itself. However, a positive outlook can add a lot to your life's journey.

For my part, I've made a decision to wake up happy and stay happy unless there is a legitimate reason not to be. (To help with that plan, I don't check the news until I've had at least one cup of coffee.) I've learned even to be happy with moments of unhappiness. While some of my optimism is an inherited trait, the rest of it is a conscious effort. It's a choice I can make every day ... and I choose the habit of being happy.

10 Small Steps to Your Happy Place

Every day ...

❶ Say "thank you" as often as possible.

❷ Wear a smile (or at least a half smile) as your default expression.

❸ Laugh out loud—and seek the people, books, and movies that get you giggling.

❹ Keep your expectations realistic.

❺ Go outdoors.

❻ Turn up the tunes and sing or dance along.

❼ Spend a few minutes practicing mindfulness meditation.

❽ Roll with your feelings—remember that they aren't permanent.

❾ Speak kindly to yourself (and everyone else).

❿ Give someone a hug, and then give one to yourself.

SMALL STEPS TOWARD ...

Habitual Happiness

As I mentioned earlier, my mantra for aging is "We can't control getting older, but we *can* control how we do it." And that applies to how I approach happiness, too. While it's true that genetics can predispose us to optimism or pessimism, and life events can influence our minute-by-minute emotions, we can still make choices to take charge of our overall attitude and life experience.

INSTEAD OF WEARING YOUR GRUMPY FACE ALL DAY,

Smile at everyone you see. Even if you're not feeling cheery at the moment, just looking the part will nudge you into a better mood. Smiling releases endorphins, which relax our muscles, reduce pain, and suppress the stress hormone cortisol. And you'll feel a much stronger sense of belonging when you see your smile reflected back at you from others.

INSTEAD OF DEMANDING PERFECTION FROM YOURSELF,

Treat yourself with patience and compassion. Self-love is essential to happiness—but many of us have developed the habit of beating ourselves up over perceived failures instead of focusing on the good things we've accomplished. Talk to yourself the way you would to a beloved friend: With kind words and affection, not harsh criticism. When something goes wrong, tell yourself, "It's okay. This is a really difficult situation, and I'm doing the best that I can."

INSTEAD OF FOCUSING ON THINGS YOU DON'T LIKE,

Compliment somebody. Turn your attention outward and bring a moment of joy to a friend or stranger with a word of praise. Odds are good that if you make another person glow, you'll feel good, too. Another benefit? People who have been complimented will be more likely to compliment someone else, creating a chain of good feelings.

INSTEAD OF SHOPPING FOR YOURSELF,

Buy a gift for someone else. If you really need some retail therapy, make it count. People who spend money on others instead of themselves feel happier afterward—especially if the gift is tied to gratitude, rather than a specific occasion. And remember: It doesn't have to be expensive, just thoughtful.

INSTEAD OF TRYING TO REMEMBER ALL THE BLESSINGS IN YOUR HEAD,

Jot them down. Buy a beautiful journal that you'll want to use. Then keep a running list of all the things for which you are grateful. Add to it often. The best part? On days when you're less than happy, you'll be able to peek into your treasure trove of gratitude—and smile.

INSTEAD OF LASHING OUT,

Practice empathy. Nobody can live up to your expectations all the time, whether it's your spouse or the supermarket cashier. Take a few deep breaths to regain perspective, and remember that every story has two sides. If you're frustrated, count to 10 before you say anything. If there are bigger issues at play, wait for a quiet moment to discuss the situation ... and be sure to listen, not just scold.

INSTEAD OF CRITICIZING,

Listen and be respectful. Whether at home or at work, when we hear harsh criticism, our levels of cortisol rise, making us more sensitive and reactive, rather than cooperative and helpful. A much kinder—and more productive—way to manage any situation is to ask what's going on, listen to the explanation, and then offer respectful suggestions or calmly state your own needs. This approach isn't just more effective; it will also reduce your own stress and add to your feelings of happiness.

INSTEAD OF ALWAYS BEING "TOO BUSY" TO HELP OTHERS,

Say yes once in a while. Offering your time as a volunteer—whether with a formal organization or just by helping a neighbor with chores—has been proven to make good feelings soar. But there is a point of diminishing returns. If you end up overcommitted, you'll be unhappy for a whole different reason.

INSTEAD OF REPLAYING BAD MEMORIES,

Bring the good stuff into focus. We can train our brains to emphasize positive memories and downplay the negative ones. It's a matter of shifting the focus and creating your own mental movie. It takes practice, but eventually happy thoughts will become your default. First, just try to catch yourself when you're replaying negative memories. Then work on redirecting your thoughts to a good place.

INSTEAD OF SUCCUMBING TO NEGATIVITY WHEN THE GOING GETS ROUGH,

Remember how strong you really are. Having a reserve of happiness allows you to shore up your resilience so you can handle difficult situations more effectively and successfully. Take good care of your physical self and develop the habits of gratitude, kindness, patience, self-love, and positivity now so that you can maintain a healthy perspective when things go wrong.

INSTEAD OF GETTING DISTRACTED BY THE PAST OR FUTURE,

Experience the beauty of now. When you are completely immersed in the here and now, that focus is like a shield, protecting you from pointless worry and regret.

INSTEAD OF KEEPING A STIFF UPPER LIP,

Share your feelings. While women tend to discuss their emotions more often than men, we often hesitate when we're in a real crisis, not wanting to "bother" anybody. But sharing feelings and allowing other people to help us once in a while is actually a way of strengthening relationships and releasing negative emotions that could otherwise make us sick. If you don't feel comfortable talking about something with friends or family, seek out a counselor or life coach. But don't keep it bottled up.

INSTEAD OF FEELING HOPELESS,

Take control and do something. It's hard to stay positive when you feel overwhelmed by external circumstances, but one of the best ways to take back the reins is to act.

Don't slide into passivity. Instead, make a plan and put it into motion. Even if all you do is list possible actions, it will help you feel more proactive and less hopeless.

INSTEAD OF LETTING YOUR MOOD DRAG YOU DOWN,

Get some exercise. Engaging in physical activity will not only add to your overall health and well-being; it will also release hormones that can quickly improve your mood (especially if you really exert yourself).

INSTEAD OF MULTITASKING,

Do one thing at a time. Focus completely on the act of driving, reading, cooking, or whatever it is you're doing. This is especially important when talking with other people. Don't check your phone while having discussions—or while the grocery clerk is ringing up your purchase. Give each person your full attention, and expect the same in return. When you're being mindful, each activity you engage in adds more pleasure to your life. *Bonus:* You make fewer mistakes, too.

INSTEAD OF WOLFING DOWN MEALS,

Savor every bite. If we rush through our meals, eating while driving, standing, or even walking, it's bad for our digestion and our sense of contentment. Instead, sit down and enjoy every meal. Turn off the television and devices and focus on the flavors and textures of each bite. *Bonus:* By eating more slowly, you may eat less.

INSTEAD OF STRESSING ABOUT CLUTTER,

Get rid of it. Being surrounded by too much stuff you don't want can add frustration and anxiety to your environment. Set aside a weekend to purge, and recycle or donate things that no longer fit into your life. And don't collect more!

INSTEAD OF SWEATING OVER BILLS,

Live below your means. Money is one of the biggest stressors for many people— and the cause of a significant number of relationship problems and divorces. One of the fastest ways to add to your happiness is simply to spend less and save more. Sounds hard, but if you take an honest look at your expenses, you'll likely discover you're spending money on things that aren't necessary and don't make you any happier. Cut them out and feel your stress levels sink.

INSTEAD OF PROCRASTINATING,

Get the information you need, then just do it. We rob ourselves of energy, time, and even space when we spend too long fretting over the perfect course of action. As the saying goes, 90 percent of clutter is procrastination, including the clutter in your brain. Take action and move on.

INSTEAD OF COMPARING YOURSELF TO OTHERS (OR YOUR YOUNGER SELF),

Enjoy being who you are now. By now, we have decades of experience being ourselves and we still have many years left to enjoy the women we've become. Accept your faults, celebrate your strengths, and let yourself finally relax into your own skin.

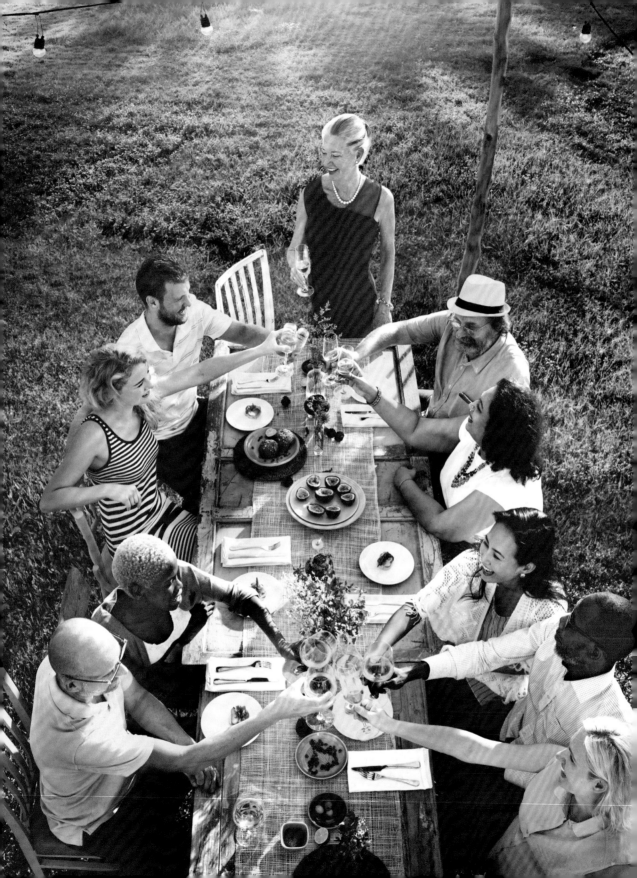

CHAPTER 13

No Woman Is an Island

"Many people will walk in and out of your life—but only true friends leave footprints in your heart."

—ELEANOR ROOSEVELT

Most women thrive on the building and nourishing of friendships, and as we get older, we rely on these essential relationships as a support system to help us navigate the topsy-turvy changes in our lives, like menopause, career shifts, divorces, new marriages, kids leaving home (or coming back), illnesses, deaths, aging parents, financial upheavals, and so much more.

And it works! As scientific studies and anecdotal evidence have shown, people with the strongest social networks have the easiest time adapting to all kinds of changes. What's more, they are measurably healthier, and—big bonus—they live longer, too.

- According to a study conducted at Brigham Young University, people with strong social connections have a 50 percent higher rate of survival than those with few social ties.

- A longitudinal study done by the Centre for Ageing Studies at Flinders University in South Australia discovered that a circle of friends could prolong an individual's life even more than close family relatives. In fact, those who had a tight-knit circle of friends lived 22 percent longer than those who did not!

- The ongoing Nurses' Health Study, managed by Harvard Medical School, has found significant evidence that women with strong social networks are less likely to develop physical disabilities as they get older. The results of the study were so powerful that the researchers described the lack of close friends as being "as detrimental to your health as smoking or carrying extra weight."

66 *The only way to have a friend is to be one."*

—RALPH WALDO EMERSON

- Reaching out to friends may strengthen two structures in your brain responsible for psychological well-being, according to a 2015 study from researchers at the University of Texas at Austin.

- Studies show that staying socially engaged stimulates the brain in areas critical to learning and memory.

The benefits of a strong social network may be one reason that women live longer than men. Social scientists around the world have studied patterns of behavior among each group and concluded that having a supportive circle of friends and family around them—through good times and bad—helps women to better cope with all kinds of stress. Men tend to keep their worries and problems to themselves while women are more likely to reach out to others (especially girlfriends), which helps us to reduce stress—and reduce stress-related illnesses. This may also partly explain why married men tend to have better health and longer lives than bachelors: They can rely on their wives for emotional support and companionship.

Tend and Befriend

A UCLA study published in 2000 showed that women are biologically adapted to help each other through

Can You Put a Price on Friendship?

Well, no, because for most of us, our meaningful relationships are priceless. But in a study published in 2008 in the *Journal of Socio-Economics,* researchers estimated the financial equivalence of either strengthening or weakening social ties. Their findings?

- An active social life can boost your life satisfaction by the equivalent of an extra $130,000 a year.

- A happy marriage is worth roughly $105,000 in additional annual income.

- Seeing friends and family regularly gives you almost another $100,000 in take-home happiness.

LOVE YOUR AGE

difficult times. How? When a woman is stressed, her body releases the hormone oxytocin, which squashes the more primal fight-or-flight response and instead triggers "tend-and-befriend" behaviors that cause us to seek nurturing social contact—especially with our children and other women. During these interactions, our bodies release even more oxytocin, which further counters stress and produces a calming effect.

Shock Value

According to a University of Virginia study, the brain scans of people who were told their friends would get an electric shock registered the same way as the scans they had when told the shock would happen to them. Now that's empathy!

Unfortunately for the guys, this response doesn't happen in men. Researchers suspect that testosterone—which men produce in higher levels than we do, especially when they're under stress—reduces the effects of oxytocin. Estrogen, on the other hand, seems to enhance it.

A Family of Friends

Being engaged with family is an important part of staying emotionally and physically active as we get older. Family relationships tend to be mutually supportive, and they keep us in touch with both past and future generations. But although these powerful bonds are biologically structured, they still need attention and nurturing to stay strong.

What's more, while many of us treasure the connections with our close relatives, others do not. In these cases, we can still get the same sense of belonging by relying on friends and more distant relatives to create our own "family of choice."

And many of us do. According to a study from the University of Oxford, almost 60 percent of those who participated said friends are the most important thing in their lives—above money, career, and, yes, family.

The Japanese have a term for the people in our lives who are committed to our happiness and well-being, and we to theirs: *kenzoku,* which means "family." The kenzoku ties aren't necessarily blood bonds but are so powerful that time and distance do nothing to diminish them. Of my eight closest girlfriends, only three of them are related to me—my sister and two cousins—but I know all of them will always have my back, even if we sometimes bicker. That's why they are permanent members of my "kenzoku circle."

Whether related by blood or affection, we all need people in our lives who love us as we are. Because when things seem darkest, turning to someone who understands you—without needing to explain yourself—is a true blessing.

Lovers for Life

While spouses and life partners don't influence our longevity quite as much as a supportive circle of girlfriends—it's surprising but true!—they are obviously important to our lives. And a 2016 study from Michigan State University found that especially for couples over 50, having a happy spouse is strongly linked to better health as we age.

But the older we get, the more likely it becomes that marriages and romantic relationships will change, too. Some will end, of course, whether due to death or divorce, but even the longest-lasting relationships can be rocked when the kids finally move out, leaving us alone together for the first time in decades; when one of us changes careers or retires; when we have to take care of our own aging parents—or when one of us gets sick. So it's important to nurture these relationships as our situations change.

Hugging: The Friendly Immunity Booster

Giving a hug is a great way to express love—but it might also keep you healthy. In 2014 researchers at Carnegie Mellon University monitored more than 400 people and found that those who had the most loving social interactions sailed through an infection with fewer symptoms. What's more, researchers calculated that of the many types of social support participants received, physical affection like hugging and touching was responsible for 32 percent of the immune-boosting effect!

SOME KEYS TO A HAPPILY EVER AFTER?

Keep your expectations reasonable. Remember the secret to happiness? It's true for relationships, too. Don't expect your partner to be someone they aren't, and don't ask them for things they can't provide, whether it's mind reading, fashion advice, or a heart-to-heart conversation during a playoff game.

Communicate. Whether you've been together for 20 years or 20 months, the ability to communicate honestly and clearly is the core of any successful relationship. Say what you mean, and mean what you say. Got an issue that needs resolving? Think it through on your own first to clarify what you want and what your partner can (realistically) do to help, then discuss it without drama or finger-pointing.

Empathize. Sure, you love your partner, but you're still different people. When there's conflict or when you don't understand why they keep doing that thing that makes you crazy, consider their side of the situation, not just your own. A little compassion goes a long way in any relationship.

Do things together—and apart. Make a point of sharing activities you both enjoy, whether it's something new you can learn together or an old favorite you haven't pursued since before the kids were born. But also pursue separate interests and see your own friends. No one person can meet all of our relationship needs, and constant together time can fray even the strongest ties.

Show affection. The happiest couples are generally the ones who are most comfortable giving and receiving affection, especially physical touch. Sex is a great way to keep the love alive, of course, but kissing, hugging, or even holding hands will release oxytocin and other hormones that help you feel connected. And don't overlook the relationship-boosting power of a cheery text message or a love note on the fridge.

Furry Friends Count, Too!

Many studies have found that owning a pet can reduce depression and stress—and just petting an animal can lower blood pressure almost instantly. A 2011 review published in the *Journal of Personality and Social Psychology* revealed that pet owners had higher measures of self-esteem and well-being than people who didn't own pets, and concluded that pets can serve as important sources of emotional support for their owners.

Of course, pet ownership is a long-term commitment. If you're an animal lover but your lifestyle doesn't lend itself to keeping a pet, there are still plenty of ways to engage with the fur brigade. Offer to dog-sit for a neighbor, foster a kitten for a few weeks, or volunteer regularly at a local animal shelter or stable.

Alone Time or Lonely Time?

While friends are critical to our well-being, most of us also benefit from regular downtime to reconnect with our inner best bud.

However, a 2014 poll conducted by AOL and the *Today* show found that over 40 percent of women say they fear being alone. If you're one of them, the challenge is to learn how to benefit from your time alone, and not let it morph into unhealthy feelings of isolation.

Part of the difference involves choice: If you control how much and how often you're alone, you're more likely to view it as a positive rather than feeling abandoned or ignored. But mostly it comes down to self-acceptance: If you know and love yourself, you'll probably enjoy your own company and the time to do your own thing, but if you don't, you'll be more likely to want to distract yourself with the stimulation of other people—even if you don't like them all that much.

FIVE GREAT REASONS TO SPEND MORE TIME ALONE

Selfishness is delicious. You get to do whatever *you* want to do, without worrying about other people's needs or opinions.

Creativity boost. A little solitude can help clear your mind, giving it a rest from external demands and opening it up to inspiration.

Connecting with yourself. Being alone lets you get to know yourself better, giving you a chance to remember what your own priorities are and giving you the mental space to think, dream, and plan. Besides, if you learn to be happy on your own, you'll be much less likely to put up with unhealthy relationships.

Time to rest and recharge. Getting away from other people lets your mind relax completely.

The Seven-Year (Friendship) Itch

There's an old saying that if a friendship lasts longer than seven years, it will likely last a lifetime. And according to unscientific surveys, that's about right. Most relationships—of any kind—don't last more than seven years, simply because people change over time, and friendships often peter out as we lose the things we had in common. So if you and your BFF have hung together for eight or more years, you probably really will be best friends forever.

You can experiment. If you're curious about a new sport, hobby, or recipe but aren't ready to go public, you can build up your confidence on your own before bringing in an audience.

Loneliness Busters

While spending time alone is a good thing, too much of it—especially if it isn't at our choosing—can backfire, leaving us feeling isolated and depressed. Humans, after all, evolved to be social, and our brains require the stimulation of other people from time to time. In fact, a neuroscientist at the University of Chicago has demonstrated that extended feelings of isolation can actually lead to lower cognitive performance. (Simply being alone isn't a problem; it's the feeling of isolation that negatively impacts our brains.) An AARP study showed that people who experience feelings of loneliness are less likely to be involved in activities that build social networks, such as volunteering, spending time on hobbies, or attending religious services.

So if you find yourself feeling more "sad and lonely" than "blissfully alone," try these five great ways to bring your world back into balance:

Play catch-up. Call someone you haven't spoken to in a while—especially someone who can be counted on to make you laugh. Or check in with an older relative, who might need to talk even more than you do. Even just writing a letter or an email can help you feel more connected.

Help someone else. Call, visit, or run errands for someone who is sick, elderly, suffering a loss, or working through difficult circumstances. It'll cheer you both up.

Volunteer. Join a gardening group at a local park, volunteer at a hospital, or sort books at the town library. Just make a regular commitment to get out in the world and do something that makes you feel useful and needed.

Throw an impromptu party. Invite some family and friends over for a home-cooked meal, cocktails and appetizers, or just popcorn and a movie. Don't sweat the details or go crazy decorating or planning a menu. Just make it happen as impromptu fun!

Take a kid out on the town. Want to be a hero to all ages? Offer to babysit the kid (or kids) of friends or family for an afternoon. Got kids of your own? The more, the merrier. Go to a movie, museum, or amusement park—and tap into your inner child along the way!

Social Media: To Friend or Unfriend?

One of the most wonderful things about the Internet is that we can make meaningful connections with people we might never meet face-to-face. My own network has grown exponentially as I've connected to like-minded women online. They enlighten, motivate, inspire, and engage me every day. Social media can help us find others who share our interests and can help us keep up with loved ones far away. So it's no

Blanketed in Love

One of women's greatest strengths and joys in life is building strong connections, creating lasting bonds that I envision as a great big cozy blanket we knit together as we forge ahead in life.

And, speaking of cozy blankets, one of the best things I've ever done was to start a Knit-a-Hug group in my neighborhood. We meet every week to knit, crochet, laugh, chat, have a glass of wine, and connect in ways that our busy lives would not otherwise allow. Some of our handiwork goes to family and friends, but we often create things that go to people we'll never meet who are in need and could use a nice, warm lovingly stitched hug.

Not a knitter? Consider organizing a book club, quilting circle, gardening gang, or even just a monthly potluck with some friends. Having a standing weekly or monthly commitment—especially one with a purpose—will encourage you to make time to get together. And if you find a way to give back to your community at the same time, that'll make you feel even better.

surprise that one of social media's fastest growing user groups in the United States is women over 45.

However, if we spend too much time online—and especially if the connections we make there are weak or superficial—it can prevent us from having more meaningful interactions in person. The result? We may end up feeling even more isolated and alone. So, what to do?

Strike a balance.

Carve out a little time once a day to check in with social media, but allocate even more time to your real-life BFFs. And in all of your relationships, go for quality over quantity. Even if you only ever communicate with someone via online messages, you can still share thoughtful conversations and real emotions. And these are the kind of connections we all crave.

Shed a Friend, Improve Your Life

As important as close friends are, there are some people who are "friends" in name only.

In her book *You Gotta Have Girlfriends,* Suzanne Braun Levine explains that most of us need to break up with a toxic friend at some point in our lives: "There are those we called friends who are now and always were unhealthy—belittling our achievements, dismissing our concerns, being disloyal—but somehow became embedded in our lives," she observes. "They drag us down, hold us back, or just don't understand (or don't care to understand) what is going on. They must go."

We've all had friends like these, and I'm sure we've held on to the relationships for valid reasons ... until these reasons no longer make sense. There's something magical about getting older that makes us want to simplify, declutter, and pare back our lives. We also want to be—and should be—around people who genuinely want the best for us, and are there to support us when we hurt. Of course, we should have always wanted relationships with those who bring us joy. But by this time of our lives, we're finally fearless enough to make it happen.

Friendship by the Numbers

In one lifetime, an individual forms approximately 396 friendships—but only one in 12 of these relationships ends up lasting many years. And only about six of these pals are considered "close" friends, while the others are "social" friends.

How to end a toxic relationship depends on your personality and the circumstances.

You can either let it die slowly by avoiding contact, or you can choose to say—in person, by phone, or in writing—that you don't think the two of you are a good match anymore. If you just don't have much in common, it's fair to say so and give the relationship a polite closure. But if the "friend" in question has a history of manipulating you despite what you want, it's probably best to let it fade quietly away rather than open yourself up to another round.

Friendships: They Can Change Your Life

Life is busy even during the calmest of times, and you can always invent a reason why you don't have time to see a friend, or go out and meet new people. But cultivating close relationships reaps many benefits, especially as we get older. The human brain, which is just 2 percent of our total body weight, gobbles up 20 percent of our body's energy. One reason may be that whenever we have downtime, our brain immediately starts strategizing on how to make social connections rather than conserving energy by just hanging out. Scientists have observed that whenever the human brain has even a few minutes to relax, the "go social" switch gets turned on, triggering us to look for companionship.

10 Small Steps to a Lifetime of Friendships

❶ Make time for relationships, even if you have to schedule them.

❷ Savor alone time just as much as friend and family time.

❸ Learn to listen more and talk less.

❹ Give help when asked, and ask for help when you need it.

❺ Practice compassion throughout the day.

❻ Hug, and hug some more.

❼ If you love someone, show it.

❽ If a relationship doesn't bring you joy, let it go.

❾ Welcome new people into your social circle as the years go on.

❿ Seek ways to build community starting within your home and working outward.

Staying Connected Now, So We Can Age Better Later

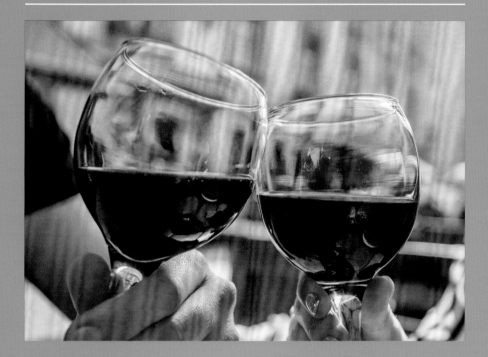

If friends can make us so much happier and healthier, why is it so hard to find time to be with them? Here are some simple ideas for boosting your social life—and your well-being, too:

INSTEAD OF EATING ALONE,

Invite someone to join you. Eating lunch with favorite co-workers gives you a midday social break—even if that means sharing your brown bags on a park bench. Instead of dinner for one, make one of your comfort-food specialties and invite a neighbor over. Plan a potluck dinner with friends once a week and share the meal prep.

INSTEAD OF PROMISING TO "CATCH UP SOON,"

Make a standing date and don't break it. As we've learned, friends and social experiences are critical to our happiness, health—and possibly even our longevity. So let's put our personal relationships where they belong: front and center. Set up regular get-togethers with your closest friends and prioritize them over life's nagging demands.

INSTEAD OF ACCUSING OTHERS OF NOT BEING THERE FOR YOU,

Focus on being present for other people. True friendship is a reciprocal relationship and doesn't involve scorekeeping.

INSTEAD OF FRETTING OVER WHAT PEOPLE THINK OF YOU,

Get interested in other people. If you feel anxious in social settings, turn your attention outward. This is especially helpful for introverts, but all of us can benefit by asking more questions—and listening to the answers. Meeting new people and making new connections allows you to expand your horizons, gain new insights, and build confidence. And don't underestimate the icebreaker potential of simply confessing that you feel awkward. You probably aren't the only one.

INSTEAD OF HIDING AT HOME BECAUSE YOU DON'T LIKE CROWDS,

Make a date for one-on-one time. You don't have to choose between loud parties and a deserted island. Many of us thrive on quality time with just one or two other people. Invite an acquaintance to join you for a museum visit or grab coffee once a week with a colleague.

INSTEAD OF SOCIALIZING ONLY WITH PEOPLE YOUR OWN AGE,

Seek out older and younger generations, too. People of different ages have different life experiences and perspectives, and they all make our lives richer. If you have children and older relatives, make time for all of them. If not, jump on opportunities to share company with people in different life stages than yourself. Invite an elderly neighbor for dinner, or that young couple from down the street. Volunteer in an elementary school or at a senior center or take a class in an activity that caters to people outside your generation.

INSTEAD OF WORRYING THAT YOU DON'T FIT IN,

Find your tribe. Pursue your own interests and seek out classes, clubs, and organizations focused on the things that you care about. You'll meet new people who can inspire you and reinforce your sense of purpose and belonging.

INSTEAD OF AVOIDING OUTINGS TO SAVE MONEY,

Invite friends to join you in cheap thrills. If you have friends in higher income brackets, you might feel left out of pricy get-togethers. But most of us just want to spend time together, not spend money for the sake of it. So keep your eye out for less expensive events—concerts in the park, affordable lunch spots, free lectures at the library or museum—and pull your posse together to join you.

INSTEAD OF CUTTING YOURSELF OFF AFTER A CONFLICT,

Be the first to apologize. True, constant bickering may indicate a toxic relationship. But if you've had a petty one-time argument with a friend or family member whose company you otherwise value, just own up to your role in the fight and move on. After all, friendship is a cooperative effort, not a zero-sum game.

INSTEAD OF RELYING ON ONE PERSON
TO BE THERE FOR YOU ALL THE TIME,

Be a reliable friend to as many other people as possible. This works two ways. It's impossible for one person to be everything to someone else, so we all need a wide web of support. And by doing your part to support other people, you'll take your mind off yourself and will broaden your social network enough so that when you do need help, you'll have a greater variety of people ready and able to give it.

INSTEAD OF USING YOUR FAMILY
AND FRIENDS AS THERAPISTS,

Go to professionals. Your friends and family can't—and shouldn't—be your medical and mental support system. It's okay to vent to them once in a while if they're willing to listen, but when it comes to serious—or frequent—stressors, doctors and specialists have the training, knowledge, and experience to help you diagnose and treat your problems. Asking your loved ones to fulfill these roles won't help you and isn't fair to them.

INSTEAD OF WISHING YOU HAD THE FAMILY YOU WANT,

Create a family of friends. Not all families are biological. Celebrate life's joys, and work through the sorrows, with the people who matter to you, regardless of how they came into your life.

INSTEAD OF AVOIDING RELIGION ALTOGETHER,

Find a spiritual community that suits you. According to a 2014 study, people who attend religious services weekly are 17 percent more likely to feel "very happy" than those who don't attend. Seek out a religious organization or spiritual center that aligns with your beliefs, and go regularly. If you're nonreligious, consider attending a meditation center or joining a humanist society. Not only will it feed your soul, it will keep you connected to a community of people who watch out for each other.

INSTEAD OF WORKING OUT ALONE,

Ask for company. Whether you're starting a new exercise routine or recommitting to an old one, invite a friend or two to join you. You'll be more likely to stick with your good habits if you're accountable to someone else—and you'll get a social boost, too.

INSTEAD OF BEING YOUR OWN WORST ENEMY,

Become a true friend to yourself. Loving who you are, showing kindness and compassion for yourself, and taking care of your body, mind, and spirit are the first steps toward being a good friend to others.

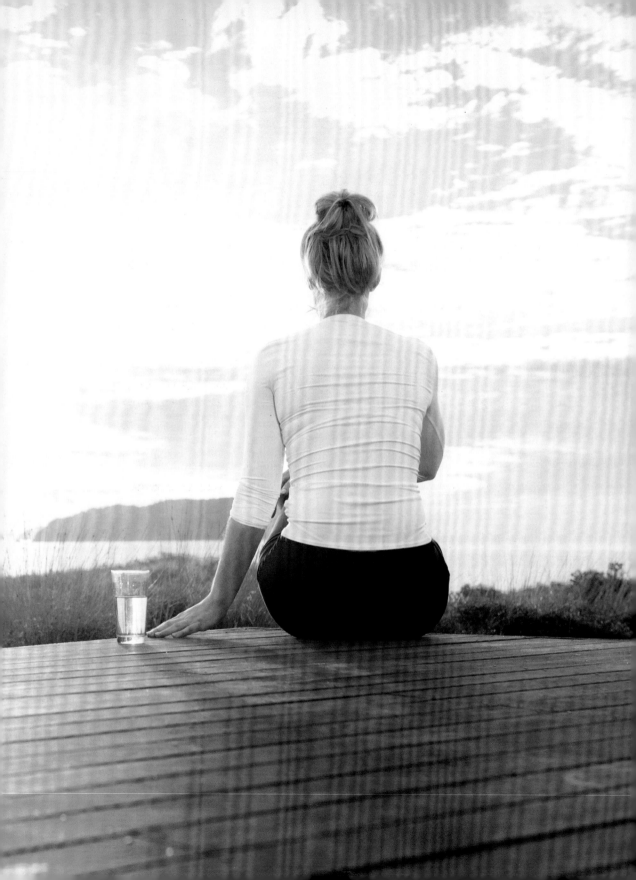

CHAPTER 14

No One Wants to Talk About ...

"Women are put in a position of feeling embarrassed about their bodies. It's so ridiculous, but also astounding."

—YOKO ONO

You know those things you worry about but don't want to discuss? Not even with your best buddies or your doctor? Those things you stress about and possibly even lose sleep over?

That's what we're going to talk about.

And why don't we talk about them? Two reasons: Either they make us feel embarrassed, or they make us think of the A-word (yes: aging).

So let's drop the drama and start the discussion. Yes, our bodies change as we get older. It's normal! Most of these changes are no big deal. But sometimes they can throw us for a loop, making us feel like we're outcasts as we wonder, "Why me?"

But don't! Because you're not alone! We're all in this together.

Some of these "taboo topics" might require a chat with a doctor or a good old-fashioned tête-à-tête with a close friend. But all of them demand an honest and loving talk with the most important person in your life: you.

Make a habit of tackling your problems head on. And keep this in mind: Even the most frustrating problem has a solution, although you might have to take it in small steps. But these steps are worth taking, because your best life is just beginning! So don't let a few inconvenient truths get in the way of enjoying it.

A Better, Happier You

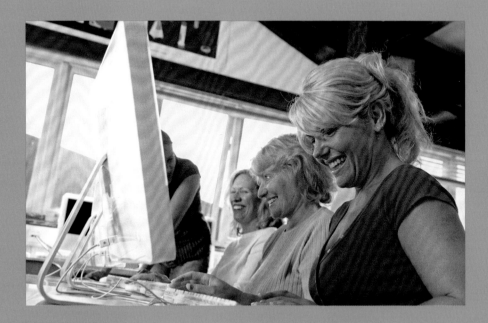

INSTEAD OF PRETENDING YOU STILL HEAR EVERYTHING,

Get your hearing tested. Hearing loss is on the rise—perhaps from all those rock concerts over the years. If you need a hearing aid, get one now and get back to your life. The newer devices are better and more discreet than ever, and the longer you wait, the harder problems will be to treat. Besides, you'll be in good company: Jodie Foster, Rob Lowe, Halle Berry, and Pete Townshend are among the many celebs who wear well-hidden hearing aids. *(See Chapter 1.)*

INSTEAD OF SQUINTING AT PRINT THAT SEEMS TO GET SMALLER AND SMALLER,

Get an eye exam. Then go buy yourself a cool pair of readers and make them a fashion statement. If you already wear prescription glasses or contacts for distance, consider getting progressive lenses to bring everything back into focus. *(See Chapter 9.)*

INSTEAD OF DENYING THAT YOU SNORE,

See a sleep specialist. Snoring can be caused by many culprits, including sleep apnea, medication, or too much alcohol. It's true that people tend to snore more often—and more loudly—as they get older, but there's usually a cause. Get it checked and get it fixed. You'll sleep more soundly, too. *(See Chapter 4.)*

INSTEAD OF GETTING FLUSTERED WHEN YOU LOSE YOUR KEYS, GLASSES, OR FORGET SOMEONE'S NAME,

Practice memory tricks. Put your keys in the same place every day, designate a landing pad for your glasses and purse, and try to associate a person's name with something else to make it easier to remember. If you have frequent episodes of "brain fog," see your doctor. Memory lapses can be caused by medications, stress, lack of sleep, or a vitamin B_{12} deficiency. If you have particular trouble remembering names or other things you've been told, get your hearing checked. Most important, to keep your brain sharp for the long term, be sure to exercise daily. *(See Chapter 7.)*

INSTEAD OF FEELING BLUE IF YOUR KIDS HAVE FLOWN THE COOP,

Find out who you are, Mama Hen. Turn this new phase of your life into an opportunity to experience the world without kids. Besides, with video chats, email, and texting, no one is ever that far away. *(See Chapter 12.)*

INSTEAD OF BEING EMBARRASSED THAT YOU'RE NOT CURRENT WITH THE LATEST TECHNOLOGY,

Take a class. Community colleges, public libraries, and tech stores often offer classes in basic computer and smartphone skills, and there are books and online tutorials for almost any tech topic. Or hire a high school or college student to teach you the ropes. Got a tech guru in your own house? Drop the ego and ask for help. Once you understand how the Internet and social media work, you can use them to stay more engaged and connected with your world.

INSTEAD OF AVOIDING EXERCISE, SEX, LONG MOVIES, OR BELLY LAUGHS BECAUSE YOU'RE WORRIED ABOUT A LEAKY BLADDER,

Find out why you're leaking. More than 40 percent of women over 40 have a sensitive bladder, which can lead to leaks. And women are more prone to leakage if they are overweight, have had babies, or have gone through menopause. Addressing the cause of your leaks is important in reducing them, so visit your doc at the first signs of trouble. In order to reduce the risk, get in the habit of emptying your bladder more often and doing Kegel exercises every day to strengthen the pelvic-floor muscles. If you're having problems, make sure you always wear the right protection, such as liners, pads, and disposable underwear specifically geared to bladder leaks so you can keep on living your life. *(See Chapter 5.)*

INSTEAD OF SKIPPING THE SHORTS IN SUMMER BECAUSE OF SPIDER VEINS,

Get them zapped. Spider veins can be caused by a number of factors, including heredity, obesity, or even a job that requires a lot of standing. If they bother you, most can be reduced or eliminated with noninvasive medical procedures, including laser treatments or sclerotherapy, which uses injections of a chemical or saline solution to close the veins. See a dermatologist to discuss your options. Or, for a quick fix, try waterproof makeup designed specifically for legs.

INSTEAD OF FREAKING OUT ABOUT FACIAL HAIRS,

Pull out the tweezers. Ever wonder why someone didn't tell you there was a long dark hair growing out of your chin? Because they won't. But the odds of sprouting an occasional facial hair go up after menopause. So mount that magnifying mirror next to a good light and double-check it before you head out the door. If the problem gets worse, consider waxing, electrolysis, or laser hair removal.

INSTEAD OF HIDING YOUR HANDS BECAUSE OF BROWN SPOTS,

Lighten them up. The gold standard for skin bleaching is dermatologist-prescribed hydroquinone, a chemical skin lightener that is generally safe and effective. However, in rare cases it can actually create dark spots on the skin, so discuss it with your dermatologist or consider other techniques, like lasers. And remember to slather the tops of your hands with sunscreen before you head outside, to prevent more spots from cropping up. *(See Chapter 10.)*

INSTEAD OF STEALING YOUR TEENAGER'S ACNE OINTMENT,

Take care of your adult skin. The good news is that as we age, the likelihood of suffering an acne outbreak is greatly reduced. Still, adult acne affects as many as 10 percent of menopausal women. Menopausal acne, also called adult-onset acne, is often deeper than the adolescent variety and tends to show up along the jawline and chin rather than in the T-zone. It is usually hereditary but may be triggered by stress, makeup, or skin-care products. If you're breaking out often, be sure that everything you put on your face is labeled "noncomedogenic" or otherwise specifies that it doesn't clog pores. Keep stress under control with good time management, regular exercise, and mindfulness practices. Eat a healthy diet without excess salt, sugar, or fat, and drink plenty of water to help flush out toxins that can upset your skin. If it doesn't clear up, a dermatologist can help treat it with topical medications matched to your specific skin conditions. *(See Chapter 10)*

INSTEAD OF SEEING RED FROM ROSACEA,

Calm it down. Over 16 million Americans suffer from rosacea, a misunderstood skin disorder often confused with allergic reactions or acne. Rosacea creates redness on the face, often with acne-like bumps and broken capillaries. People of all ages can develop rosacea, but it's especially common among midlife women, especially those with light skin. While there is no permanent cure, dermatologists can prescribe medical treatments to minimize symptoms, including topical products and laser treatments that reduce the redness and oral drugs that can help reduce outbreaks. A gentle daily facial massage can help calm the inflammation, as can avoiding common triggers such as alcohol, spicy food, and any specific cosmetic products that seem to affect your skin. You can also apply a green-tinted cosmetic foundation or CC cream to help even out your skin tone and downplay the red.

INSTEAD OF WORRYING ABOUT GAS,

Eat more fiber. Our bodies digest food more slowly as we get older, causing acid reflux, constipation, bloating, and that really embarrassing thing: flatulence. Easiest fix? Eat more fiber and drink more water to keep things moving along. However, adding too much fiber too fast can actually make the problem worse, so instead of piling on the Metamucil, start incorporating more veggies and beans into your diet a little at a time. *Other tips:* Eat at regular intervals, eat more slowly, and sip hot ginger or mint tea after your meals. Even just sipping hot water can help. *(See Chapter 3.)*

INSTEAD OF HIDING THINNING HAIR UNDER A BASEBALL CAP,

Stop thinning in its tracks. You can't easily grow back hair, but you may be able to stop or reduce thinning. See your dermatologist to determine the underlying cause and to discuss using Rogaine, Latisse, or other prescription-strength remedies. If your hair is already thinner than you'd like, work with your hairstylist to try salon tricks, like using dry shampoo to make hair look fuller and products that color the scalp the same shade as hair. And don't be afraid to try extensions or wigs—you won't believe how many stars do! *(See Chapter 11.)*

INSTEAD OF COVERING UP YOUR ARMS AND LEGS DUE TO FREQUENT BRUISES,

Strengthen your skin's natural barrier. Skin gets thinner and more fragile as we get older, resulting in easy bruising that can be even worse if you're on blood thinners. The bad news is that we can't completely prevent this, since it's a natural part of aging. But we can strengthen the skin's natural barrier by staying hydrated, by being diligent about applying moisturizing cream all over, and by wearing sunscreen to protect skin from additional sun damage. Eating a diet rich in vitamin C can help as well, as can eating plant proteins, such as soy and nuts, which contain phytoestrogens that can help slow the loss of collagen due to menopause. *(See Chapter 10.)*

INSTEAD OF WATCHING YOUR BREASTS DROOP FARTHER DOWNWARD,

Give them a lift. Most women don't wear the right bra size, and it shows. Our bodies change throughout life, and so do the size and shape of our breasts. Skin loses elasticity and, yes, breasts will start to sag—although how much depends on their size and density. Get measured and fitted for new bras at least once a year, and look for those that lift and separate. It's amazing what the right bra can do. *(See Chapter 11.)*

INSTEAD OF HIDING YOUR DEPRESSION,

Bring it into the open. Research by AARP shows that from your early 50s on, happiness increases. Still, depression is not uncommon among women over 45 for many reasons, including the hormonal upheaval from menopause and major life changes, like kids growing up and parents aging, plus coming to terms with getting older. It's no crime to feel depressed, even if you've always been the cheery one. But don't let it linger, because depression can quickly overtake your life. Grab a girlfriend and talk it out, and if that doesn't lift your spirits considerably or if you've been feeling down for more than two weeks, consider seeing a professional. *(See Chapter 12.)*

INSTEAD OF WONDERING IF THAT SECOND (OR THIRD, OR FOURTH ...) GLASS OF WINE IS TOO MUCH,

Admit that it is. Medical experts agree: Women should stick with one glass of alcohol per day—two only on occasion. Wine, particularly red wine, has its place in a healthy diet, but once you start to overimbibe, the benefits fade away. Take a look at whether drinking has become an unhealthy habit or stress reliever. If so, make a plan to break the habit and look for better ways to ease your stress. (Exercise comes to mind.) If limiting yourself to one drink a day is a challenge, talk with your doctor.

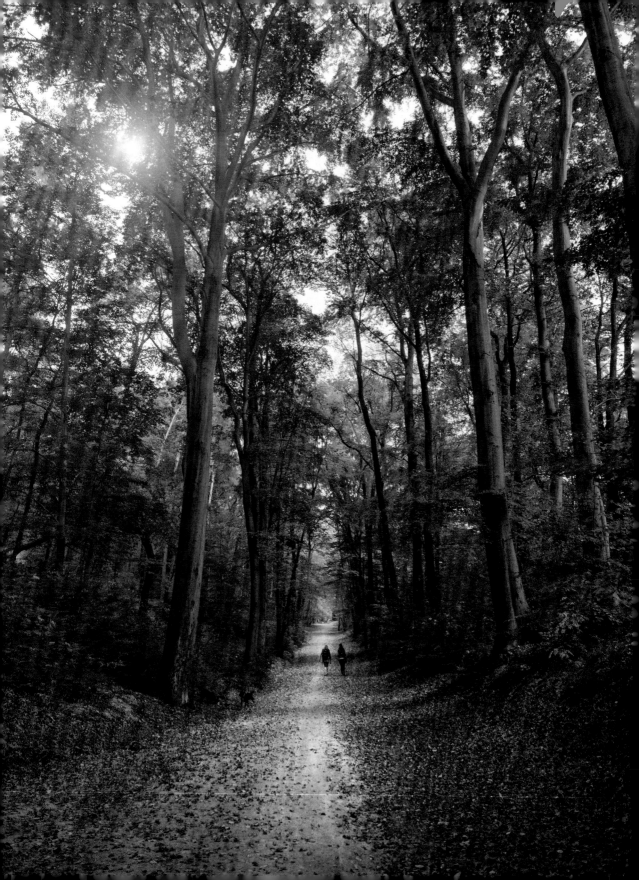

CHAPTER 15

Small Steps, Big Difference

The Master Cheat Sheet to Improve Your Life—One Step at a Time

See? You can make big changes in your life without turning it upside down. To prove it, I've pulled together the best of the best tips to give you a healthy-habit master checklist—including a few *new* ideas that were just too good not to share. Every time you check one off, your life will get a bit better. I pinkie-swear! Just remember: For medical tests and other health concerns, it's best to check with your own doctors to set the schedule that's right for you.

EVERY 10 YEARS

- See an audiologist for a hearing test (if you're under 50).
- Get a Tdap vaccine booster.
- Get a colonoscopy (starting at 50, or earlier if you have a family history of colon cancer).

EVERY FIVE YEARS

- Get your cholesterol and triglyceride levels tested.

EVERY THREE YEARS

- Get a Pap smear and HPV test.
- See an audiologist for a hearing test (if you're over 50).

EVERY TWO YEARS

- See an ophthalmologist for an eye exam (starting at age 40).

- Check to see if you need to update eyeglass or lens prescriptions (or more often if necessary).
- Get a mammogram (if you're 55 or over).
- Get a blood test to check cell counts, nutrient markers, cholesterol, blood sugar, and thyroid levels.

EVERY YEAR

- Visit your PCP for a checkup.
- Get your blood pressure checked (or more often if you have a history of high blood pressure).
- Visit your dermatologist for a skin cancer screening.
- Visit your gynecologist for a pelvic exam.
- Get a mammogram (if you're under 55).
- Get a flu shot before the end of November.
- Consider a semi-fast to boost your immune system and overall health.
- Consider whitening your teeth.
- Replace lipstick, blush, concealer, foundation, and eye shadow.
- Take a few minutes to reevaluate your makeup colors or get a professional consult.
- Replace your bras and get a professional fitting to reevaluate sizing.

EVERY SIX MONTHS

- Get a dental checkup and cleaning.
- Chat with your hairstylist about how your current style, color, and products are working for you.
- Walk through your home and remove and donate things you no longer use or need.
- Go through your closet and remove any clothes that don't fit your current body or style.

EVERY THREE MONTHS

- Check the expiration dates on medications, canned goods, and frozen goods.
- Replace your mascara and eyeliner.
- Get a professional facial.
- Check out the class listings at your local library, community college, or art center.
- Take a relaxing vacation (or staycation).

EVERY MONTH

- Measure your waist.
- Record your height.

- Do a skin exam in the mirror.
- Do a breast self-exam.
- Test your blood pressure (if you have a history of high blood pressure).
- Check your resting heart rate.
- Polish your favorite jewelry.
- Clean and polish your shoes and take them in for repair if heels or soles need replacing.
- Check your clothes to see if anything needs mending or replacing.
- Try something new.
- Volunteer your time to a good cause.

EVERY WEEK

- Clean out the produce bin in your fridge.
- Make a meal plan and a grocery list.
- Opt for whole foods instead of processed ones.
- Read the labels before you buy groceries.
- Make a pitcher of green or herbal tea.
- Try a new recipe.
- Sharpen your kitchen knives.
- Cut up some veggies and put them in the fridge for snacking.
- Cook legumes and grains, and stash them in the fridge or freezer for upcoming meals.
- Wash your makeup brushes.
- Participate in a religious service or spiritual ritual that feeds your soul.
- Spend time with friends.
- Spend some quality time with yourself.
- Scan the event listings in the local paper for interesting things to do.
- Call someone you haven't spoken to in a while.

EVERY OTHER DAY

- Cook dinner at home (more often is even better!).
- Enjoy an ounce of dark chocolate (okay, maybe do this every day).
- Brush your pet's hair.
- Wipe down your phone and computer keyboard with a disinfectant wipe.
- Exfoliate your body, face, and lips.

> **"Without friends no one would choose to live, though he had all other goods."**
>
> —ARISTOTLE

- Eat a three- to four-ounce serving of heart-healthy fish.
- Enjoy a glass of red wine with dinner (I'll give you this one on the daily, as well).
- Learn a new word.

EVERY DAY

- Make yourself the priority.
- Scan your body with your mind and take note of how you feel.
- Don't smoke (if you're quitting, take it one day at a time—and if you've never smoked, don't start!).
- Drink a glass of water first thing in the morning.
- Scrape your tongue, for better breath and oral health.
- Floss your teeth before brushing.
- Brush your teeth at least morning and night.
- Slather your body with lotion or olive oil after showering.
- Massage olive oil or cuticle cream into your cuticles.
- Dab on a dot of eye cream in the morning.
- Moisturize your face, neck, and chest.
- Apply sunscreen before you go outside.
- Curl your eyelashes before putting on mascara.
- Moisturize your lips with balm.
- Apply hand cream after washing.
- Make your bed.
- Hang up your towels.
- Clean your glasses.
- Put on a warm hat in the winter.

- Put on a sun hat in the summer.
- Put on sunglasses before you walk out the door, no matter what the weather.
- Start your day with a protein-packed breakfast.
- Drink a cup of coffee (or two) in the morning, but skip the sweetener.
- Eat a half cup of Greek yogurt.
- Pop a probiotic pill.
- Take vitamin D supplements for bone health, and B$_{12}$ if you need it.
- Eat at least three servings of veggies and two servings of fruit.
- Eat whole grains.
- Eat lean protein.
- Choose olive oil over butter.
- Serve your meals on smaller plates.
- Load your plate with vegetables, then add grains and protein.
- Drink a glass of water several times a day.
- Keep a food journal.
- Strike a Wonder Woman pose—and hold it!
- Look for opportunities to move your body as often as possible.
- Walk 10,000 steps.
- Walk a little faster.
- Exercise for at least 30 minutes—and get your heart rate up to at least 50 percent of max for 15 minutes.
- Do push-ups (10 or more), planks (as long as you can), plié squats, wall squats, and chair dips, or your fave strengthening exercises.
- If you're working at a desk, get up, walk around, and gaze into the distance every 20 minutes.
- Practice balancing throughout the day.
- Stretch or do yoga every few hours.
- Sit up straight when seated.
- Chew on a few sprigs of mint or parsley for fresh breath.
- Hug someone.
- Pet a pet.
- Wash your hands often.
- Moisturize your hands every time you wash.
- Wear rubber gloves while doing the dishes.
- Squeeze in some Kegels.
- Put down your cell phone and listen to the people in front of you.
- Smile.

- Laugh as often as possible.
- Read your daily snail mail, respond to any that needs attention, then recycle it.
- Delete spam emails.
- Do mindfulness meditation for at least five minutes.
- Write in your gratitude journal.
- Turn off the TV and other electronics at least 90 minutes before bed.
- Turn down the lights in the evening.
- Remove your makeup and wash your face one hour before bed.
- Apply a retinoid after your face dries.
- Apply night cream after retinoids.
- Turn down the thermostat to 67 (or lower) at night.
- Moisturize your feet and put on socks before bed.
- Count your blessings.
- Get at least seven hours of sleep.
- Say "I love you" to someone.
- Embrace your age.

WHEN YOU NEED A BOOST
- Go outside.
- Get moving.
- Pay someone a compliment.
- Call someone you care about.
- Smile at the next stranger you see.
- Make a list of 12 things that make you smile.
- Write a letter of gratitude to someone who did something nice for you.
- Buy a spontaneous gift for someone.
- Close your eyes and think about your favorite place.
- Remember when you were eight, think about what made you happy then—and do it.
- Eat a handful of blueberries or grapes.
- Put on some lipstick.
- Smile at yourself in the mirror.
- Lie down on the floor with your legs up the wall for five minutes.
- Turn on some music—and dance.
- Video chat with a girlfriend.
- Give yourself a pep talk.
- Breathe deeply for 10 full breaths.
- Do another plank.

WHEN SOMETHING DOESN'T SEEM RIGHT

- Trust your instincts.
- Pay attention to your body.
- Call your PCP or specialist.
- Take charge of your own health.

BEFORE GETTING PHYSICAL WITH A NEW FLAME

- Get tested for STDs—and make sure your would-be partner does the same.

WHEN YOU HAVE ONE SPARE MINUTE

- Recycle something.
- Empty your pockets, purse, and wallet of coins and save them in a jar.
- Stash a reusable bag where you'll remember to take it to the store.
- Do a one-minute "straighten-up" of one room in your house.
- Massage your head.
- Eat 10 almonds as a snack.
- Sip a cup of green tea.
- Send your love interest a flirty text.
- Plan a sexual encounter.
- Start a crossword puzzle.
- Do as many jumping jacks as you can.

WHENEVER YOU CAN

- Take the stairs.
- Say "thank you."
- Give up your seat to someone else.
- Forgive someone who's hurt you.
- Hug someone.
- Hug yourself.
- Tell a good joke (or a bad one).
- Laugh.
- Laugh some more.
- Pay yourself a compliment.
- Choose joy.

Take a small step to your best life and keep going.

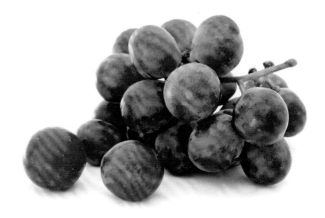

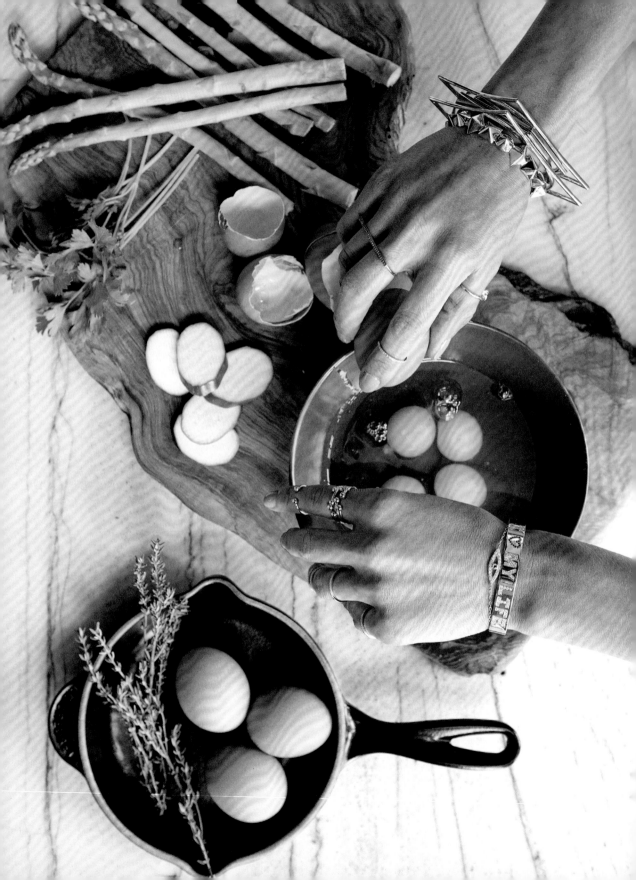

One Habit to Rule Them All

The defining characteristic of a habit is that it's almost completely involuntary. It's a thought or an action so ingrained in your psyche and life that you don't even think about it. Automation at its best!

We get up, go to the bathroom, splash water on our faces, plod into the kitchen, switch on the coffee maker, check our email, turn on the morning news … and so on. Some of us can make it a solid hour or two into our day without making a single conscious choice.

However, you can be sure that no matter how mindless it is, every one of these routine actions is shaping your life today—and far into the future. For instance, every time your daily commute takes you to the drive-through for a mochaccino, you're adding as many as 350 extra calories into your day—out of your daily recommended allocation of 1,800!—which means that you'll have a hard time maintaining your weight. You're also getting a huge shot of sugar, which will give you a jittery buzz for an hour before your blood sugar crashes, leaving you tired, unable to concentrate, and hungry for anything—healthy or not—that will fill the void. And the more often you do that, the greater the risk that you'll end up overweight or develop diabetes, which, in turn, could raise your risk of heart disease and vision problems—not to mention a much lower quality of life, and possibly premature death.

Sounds dramatic, I know, but it's true! Every choice you make has consequences— even the ones that are so habitual they don't even seem like choices anymore.

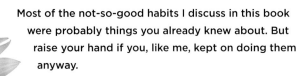

Most of the not-so-good habits I discuss in this book were probably things you already knew about. But raise your hand if you, like me, kept on doing them anyway.

Why do we do this? It's not like we forgot that these decisions are bad for us—or didn't know (or at least suspect) that other choices would be better. It's just that it's so easy to keep coasting on autopilot, right? But the small steps you take now will have a huge impact on your body and life, almost instantly.

For instance, let's flip that domino effect around. What if you swapped your daily mochaccino habit for a cup of unsweetened black coffee instead (try a tiny drop of heavy cream, like I do). You just wiped out all those negative consequences in one fell swoop! You improved your mood and productivity for the day, reduced your food cravings, kept your weight in balance, and lowered your risk of developing a debilitating disease. PS: You also just saved yourself a few bucks a day, which doesn't sound like much, but it's plenty to buy some extra servings of wholesome fruits and veggies!

Imagine what would happen if you added a second healthy habit, like walking for 15 minutes a couple of times a day, to your routine. With that addition to your life, your mood would improve, your stress would be reduced, your blood pressure would go down, your muscles would tone up, and you'd burn more calories and reduce your risk of diabetes, heart disease, cancer, and more. You'd be on a roll!

Good habits don't just happen. They take some knowledge about the consequences of your actions, which leads to understanding how the choices you make affect your overall happiness and well-being. This will then lead (I hope!) to a desire to change your behavior. Then a commitment, which becomes a plan, which becomes an action, which eventually becomes: Ta-dah! A habit.

It all may sound like a lot of work. But having followed a path of healthy habits for a few years, I can honestly say that once the benefits start to add up and build their own momentum, it's pretty easy to continue. Now that I've trained myself to always slap on sunscreen before makeup, for instance, my skin really does look better and brighter, which encourages me to keep doing it. Now that I reward myself with a small square of heart-healthy dark chocolate every night, I no longer crave sweet empty calories, which helps me keep off extra pounds. And now that I do 20 push-ups each morning before breakfast (and a few more throughout the day), my arms are lean and strong, and I feel ready to hold up the world.

But even with the benefits so clear in our minds and bodies, the many demands of life can still interfere with our commitment to maintaining our well-intentioned ways.

How do I know? Oh, trust me. I know.

Within a few years of running my first marathon—and just as I was really hitting my stride with a whole new life of healthy habits—both my mother and mother-in-law developed complicated health issues. There were appointments to be made, shopping to be done, bills to be paid, and that was just for them. I still had my business to run, articles to write, my own household to manage—with one daughter starting college and another in high school—and, oh yes, a husband with an equally demanding career who needed a little TLC once in a while, too. And did I mention a rescued dog?

With all that going on (and then some), sleep, exercise, and healthy home-cooked meals started to seem like indulgences I couldn't afford. One by one, my carefully constructed routines collapsed. After a while my posture was sagging, my clothes were squeezing, and I barely had enough energy to take care of anyone else, let alone myself. Push-ups? Nope. Running? Are you kidding? Sleep. What's that? I felt like I was 10 years older than I was!

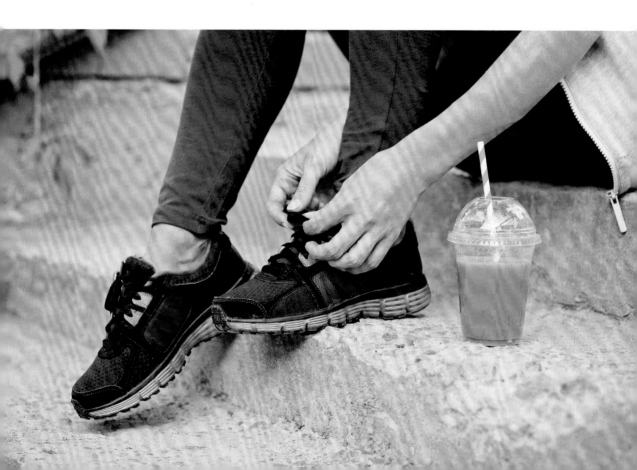

But then I remembered something the ageless fashion designer Diane von Fursten-berg once told me: "Barbara, I love my husband, kids, and grandkids unconditionally. But I love myself even more. Sound selfish? No. It's smart."

She was right, of course. People may be depending on you, but if you're not in good mental and physical shape, you won't be much use to anyone.

And that's when I realized that there really is one habit that rules them all: the habit of self-love.

Self-love—the simple act of treating ourselves as the glorious creatures we are—is the golden ticket to a happy, healthy life, regardless of what else is going on. It's the first step to every positive life change; the one habit that can corral all the others back into service; the habit that is always inside you; the one that doesn't depend on a schedule or an income or a recipe; the one you can count on when all the others skitter away. If you develop and nourish the habit of self-love, you will always have a powerful tool to put yourself back on track, at the head of the line, and in control. Because if *you* are the priority, your choices will reflect that.

So with DVF's words in mind, I brought my sorely neglected habits into my life once again. When I laced up my formerly beloved running shoes, I felt stronger and hap-pier almost immediately. Then it was just one small step after another until I was back on track.

I know there will be other phases when I will struggle to maintain my healthy routines. It will probably happen to you, too. Life is filled with bumps and twists that we can't see coming. But if you practice the habit of self-love each and every day, it will grow stronger and will always be ready to lead the way back to the life you want to be living.

But how do you get started in the first place?

You now have plenty of tools at your disposal to build the habits that will serve you for a long, lovely life. And you have knowledge, studies, heaps of research, and a plethora of medical experts ready and willing to help you along the way. All you need is to love yourself enough to honestly evaluate the habits you have now. Keep the ones that bring you health, stamina, energy, confidence, and joy—and change the ones that don't.

And if you make less-than-helpful choices sometimes, don't beat yourself up. Just summon the one habit that rules them all—self-love—and take a single small step in the only direction you want to go: forward.

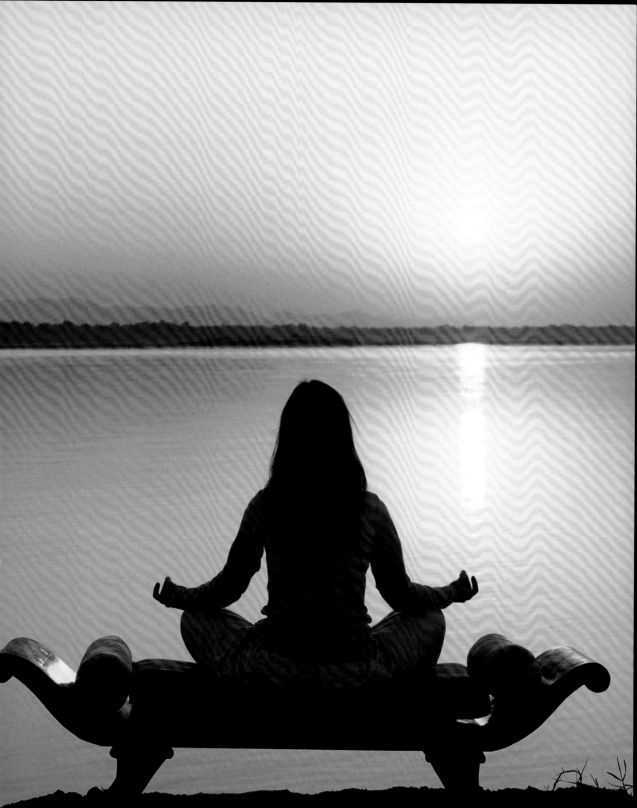

10 Small Steps to Make Those Healthy Habits Stick

---

❶ REMEMBER THE REWARDS. It's a lot easier to stay motivated if you remember why you're doing something in the first place. For instance, if you're starting a new exercise program, make a point of noticing how you feel after working out, and remind yourself of the specific benefits you're after—both short-term and long-term. I always think about how great my skin looks after I've gotten some exercise (immediate reward) and how much stronger I'll be down the road (long-term reward).

❷ TAKE BABY STEPS. Going whole hog sounds tempting when you want to change your life, but it can be overwhelming for most of us, causing us to stop before we've even started. Don't think, "If I can't do it all, I won't do anything." The small-step solution really will get you there. Just choose one or two specific actions that will improve your life (for instance: 20 push-ups or two more veggies every day) and do it consistently and regularly. Once you feel you've got that close to autopilot, choose one or two more to add to the mix … and keeping going.

❸ LET ONE LEAD THE WAY. When I chose to run and made it a regular habit, it triggered other changes over time: I slept better, ate healthier foods, and turned to specific exercises to become stronger. One healthy habit linked to another until they all started to work in tandem. But I started with just one.

❹ MAKE A PUBLIC COMMITMENT. If you want to make a change in your life, let people know. Lots of people. (Unless your daughter does it for you!) Post it on Facebook or announce it at a dinner party. Once it's "out there," it's much harder to go back. It's a mind game you can play with yourself … and always win.

❺ GIVE IT THREE MONTHS (OR 90 DAYS IF THAT SOUNDS BETTER). The only way an action can truly become a habit is when it's done regularly and consistently for however long it takes to insinuate itself into your life. For most people that's about three months. Sure, you can start to feel attached to an action in a few weeks, but the risk of giving up is much greater early on. Stay with it and the payback will be a new habit—hopefully for life.

❻ PLAN ON IT. I insert every single thing I want to do into my Google Calendar, which then gets shared on all my devices—phone, tablet, computer (even doing *this* has become a habit). Don't leave exercising, going to bed at 10 p.m., or shopping at the farmer's market for healthy veggies up to chance. Plan it, schedule it, and if it involves other people (a running buddy perhaps), send them a calendar invitation, too. And be specific: Monday, 7:00 a.m.–8:00 a.m., run.

❼ SET YOURSELF UP FOR SUCCESS. If you place your sneakers on the floor next to your bed the night before a workout, you'll be more apt to put them on. Keep the floss next to your toothbrush. Add good, healthy foods to your pantry, cabinet, and fridge, and remove as many of the "wasted-calories" foods as you can. The more you stack the deck in your favor, the better your odds of winning.

❽ COMPARE AND CONTRAST. I never used to weigh myself. But once I decided to commit to my newfound healthy life, I bought a simple scale and now weigh myself every day. It's a handy tool to track my progress and to see quick proof of what happens if I stop making good choices. Recording what you eat in a journal is proven to help create a commitment to healthy eating. And it's always motivating to compare your "before healthy habits" to "after healthy habits" with photos and journals that help you see clear evidence of the changes you've made.

❾ SET A GOAL. Maybe you dream of running your first 5K, or you want to cook a week's meals entirely from scratch. Whatever it is, having a clear goal in mind can be a powerful motivator to get you to create a life of healthy habits. For me, it all started with my daughter wanting to see me run in the New York City Marathon. And then the magic kicked in.

❿ BE #1. Put *your* needs first, including making sure that you're eating well, sleeping enough, and moving your body daily. When you are the starting point and the priority in your own life, you'll be more likely to make choices that help you feel better physically and mentally, and you'll be more open to all the other life-enhancing healthy habits that are just waiting to be embraced. It isn't selfish. It's smart.

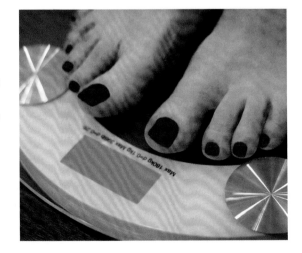

Additional Resources: Dig Deeper

Knowledge is power. To keep learning, keep reading, starting with these great resources to help you build better habits of your own.

For Overall Health

• *Being a Good Patient Can Save Your Life: A Guide to Improve Your Medical Care Now and Long Term,* Alexander L. Sytman (2014)

• *Dr. Suzanne Steinbaum's Heart Book: Every Woman's Guide to a Heart-Healthy Life,* Suzanne Steinbaum (2014)

• *Gut: The Inside Story of Our Body's Most Underrated Organ,* Giulia Enders (2015)

• *A Short Guide to a Long Life,* David B. Agus (2014)

• AARP: *www.aarp.org*

• American Heart Association: *www.americanheart.org*

• Choosing Wisely: *www.choosingwisely.org*

• Healthline: *www.healthline.com*

• Mayo Clinic Health Information: *www.mayoclinic.com*

• National Cancer Institute: *www.cancer.gov*

• National Osteoporosis Foundation: *www.nof.org*

• Office of Women's Health: *www.womenshealth.gov*

For Fitness

• *David Kirsch's Ultimate Family Wellness: The No-Excuses Program for Diet, Fitness, and Lifelong Health,* David Kirsch (2015)

• *The First 20 Minutes: Surprising Science Reveals How We Can Exercise Better, Train Smarter, Live Longer,* Gretchen Reynolds (2013)

• *No Sweat: How the Simple Science of Motivation Can Bring You a Lifetime of Fitness,* Michelle Segar (2015)

• *Strength Training Exercises for Women,* Joan Pagano (2013)

• *Women's Complete Guide to Running,* Jeff and Barbara Galloway (2011)

• Livestrong: *www.livestrong.com*

• Mile Posts: *www.mile-posts.com*

For Nutrition

• *101+ Secrets from Nutrition School,* Lynne Dorner (2014)

• *AARP New American Diet: Lose Weight, Live Longer,* John Whyte (2012)

• *The Art of Eating Well,* Jasmine Hemsley and Melissa Hemsley (2014)

• *The Blue Zones Solution: Eating and Living Like the World's Healthiest People,* Dan Buettner (2015)

• *Get the Glow: Delicious and Easy Recipes That Will Nourish You from the Inside Out,* Madeleine Shaw (2015)

• *How to Cook Everything Vegetarian,* 2nd ed., Mark Bittman (2017)

• *The New Vegetarian Cooking for Everyone,* Deborah Madison (2014)

• *The Very Best of Recipes for Health,* Martha Rose Shulman (2010)

• EatingWell: *www.eatingwell.com*

• Food Network: *www.foodnetwork .com/healthy*

For Sleep

• *Sleep Smarter: 21 Essential Strategies to Sleep Your Way to a Better Body, Better Health, and Bigger Success,* Shawn Stevenson (2016)

• *Sleep Soundly Every Night, Feel Fantastic Every Day: A Doctor's Guide to Solving Your Sleep Problems,* Robert Rosenberg (2014)

• *Thrive: The Third Metric to Redefining Success and Creating a Life of Well-Being, Wisdom, and Wonder,* Arianna Huffington (2014)

• National Sleep Foundation: *www .sleepfoundation.org*

For Menopause

• *100 Best Foods for Menopause,* Parragon Books (2015)

• *I Just Want to Be Me Again: A Guide to Thriving Through Menopause,* Jeanne D. Andrus (2015)

• *The Wisdom of Menopause: Creating Physical and Emotional Health During the Change,* Christiane Northrup (2012)

• The North American Menopause Society: *www.menopause.org*

For Sex

• *Dating After 50 for Dummies,* Pepper Schwartz (2013)

• *Getting Naked Again: Dating, Romance, Sex, and Love When You've Been Divorced, Widowed, Dumped, or Distracted,* Judith Sills (2010)

• *Mating in Captivity: Unlocking Erotic Intelligence,* Esther Perel (2007)

• *Sex After … : Women Share How Intimacy Changes as Life Changes,* Iris Krasnow (2015)

• American Sexual Health Association: *www.ashasexualhealth.org*

For Brain Health

• *5 Secrets to Brain Health,* AARP (2013)

• *100 Simple Things You Can Do to Prevent Alzheimer's and Age-Related Memory Loss,* Jean Carper (2012)

• *What You Must Know About Memory Loss & How You Can Stop It: A Guide to Proven Techniques and Supplements to Maintain, Strengthen, or Regain Memory,* Pamela Wartian Smith (2014)

• AARP's Staying Sharp program: *www.stayingsharp.org*

• Alzheimer's Association: *www.alz.org*

For Dental Health
• American Dental Association: *www.mouthhealthy.org*

• National Institute of Dental and Craniofacial Research: *www.nidcr.nih.gov /OralHealth*

For Vision Health
• *The Eye Care Revolution: Prevent and Reverse Common Vision Problems,* Robert Abel (2014)

• *Healthy Vision: Prevent and Reverse Eye Disease Through Better Nutrition,* Neal Adams (2014)

• National Eye Institute: *www.nei.nih.gov*

For Skin Care
• *Forget the Facelift: Turn Back the Clock With a Revolutionary Program for Ageless Skin,* Doris J. Day (2006)

• *Skin Rules: Trade Secrets from a Top New York Dermatologist,* by Debra Jaliman (2013)

• *A Woman's Guide to a Glowing Complexion,* by Jennifer Hamilton (2015)

• Skin Cancer Foundation: *www.skincancer.org*

For Makeup
• *Bobbi Brown Makeup Manual,* Bobbi Brown (2011)

• *Don't Go to the Cosmetics Counter Without Me,* by Paula Begoun and Bryan Barron (2012)

• *The 5-Minute Face,* Carmindy (2007)

• *Makeup Wakeup: Revitalizing Your Look at Any Age,* Lois Joy Johnson and Sandy Linter (2011)

For Style
• *How to Get Dressed: A Costume Designer's Secrets for Making Your Clothes Look, Fit, and Feel Amazing,* Alison Freer (2015)

• *How to Look Expensive: A Beauty Editor's Secrets to Getting Gorgeous Without Breaking the Bank,* Andrea Pomerantz Lustig (2012)

• *The Wow Factor: Insider Style Secrets for Every Body and Every Budget,* Jacqui Stafford (2013)

• 40+Style: *www.40plusstyle.com*

• What 2 Wear Where: *www.what2wearwhere.com*

For Happiness
• *The Happiness Advantage: The Seven Principles of Positive Psychology That*

Fuel Success and Performance at Work, Shawn Achor (2010)

• *The Happiness Project: Or, Why I Spent a Year Trying to Sing in the Morning, Clean My Closets, Fight Right, Read Aristotle, and Generally Have More Fun,* Gretchen Rubin (2009)

• *The Little Book of Mindfulness: 10 Minutes a Day to Less Stress, More Peace,* Patrizia Collard (2014)

• *Stumbling on Happiness,* Daniel Gilbert (2007)

• Tiny Buddha: *www.tinybuddha.com*

• Zen Habits: *www.zenhabits.net*

For Friendship

• *Reclaiming Conversation: The Power of Talk in a Digital Age,* Sherry Turkle (2015)

• *The Social Sex: A History of Female Friendship,* Marilyn Yalom (2015)

• *Wired to Connect: The Surprising Link Between Brain Science and Strong, Healthy Relationships,* Amy Banks and Leigh Ann Hirschman (2016)

• *You Gotta Have Girlfriends: A Post-Fifty Posse Is Good for Your Health,* Suzanne Braun Levine (2013)

Connect With Me!

Let's keep the conversation going!

There are lots of useful and actionable tips throughout this book, and plenty of additional resources you can dive into for even more information. But one of our greatest strengths and joys in life as women is our ability to learn from each other and share what we know. That's one good reason why staying connected is such a powerful tool: Together we can inspire each other to live our best lives. So let's keep the conversation going, shall we?

Join me at …

www.bestofeverythingafter50.com

• **Facebook, LinkedIn, and YouTube:**
Barbara Hannah Grufferman

• **Twitter:**
@BGrufferman

• **Instagram:**
barbarahannahgrufferman

• **Snapchat:**
Barbara Hannah Grufferman

… and help me find you too by using the hashtag #LoveYourAge in all your social media posts!

Acknowledgments

I owe so many thanks to so many people, but a few have earned particular appreciation. For their contributions, I send my superspecial, heartfelt never-ending gratitude:

• **To the many experts who have freely shared their knowledge with me via phone, email or (lucky me!) in person.** Thank you to Jeff Galloway, who helped me take the first small step into the world of running, which became the foundation of my whole new life; to Margaret Nachtigall, NYU reproductive endocrinologist and dear friend, who shared her knowledge and research so I could share it with others; to Gregory Pitaro, my PCP for over 15 years, who not only keeps me healthy but lets me pick his brain about everything medical; to Valter Longo, director of the USC Longevity Institute, who convinced me that less really is more; to Doris Day, the dermatology dynamo who taught me the secrets of great skin; to Linnea M. Duvall, kind and compassionate marriage and family therapist, who showed me the wisdom of self-love (and affirmed that talking to myself isn't crazy); to Jacqui Stafford, QVC queen and style guru, who instilled in me the confidence to embrace my body right now; to Elaine D'Farley, beauty editor and more, who makes looking fabulous easy-peasy; to Joan Pagano, fitness expert and author, who has helped me feel strong enough to hold up the world; and to the wonderful staff and dedicated board at the National Osteoporosis Foundation, where I am honored to serve as bone health ambassador and trustee.

• **To the Internet friends I've made through Facebook, Twitter, Instagram, Pinterest, and my blogs.** I am very lucky to have connected with these inspiring women! Even though I may never meet them all in person, they are an endless source of information and curiosity. They tell me what they want to know, then let me find the answers. They let me nag them about doing push-ups, and not smoking, and eating well, and eating less, and embracing their age—and they remind me there's always a reason to say "Yay!" ... no matter what life throws at us. In many ways, I wrote this book because of them, and for them.

• **To my best girlfriends, near and far.** I rely daily on our talks, walks, runs, rants, coffees, emails, texts, tears, and many bouts of uncontrollable laughter. You know who you are, and you are my kenzoku sisters for life.

• **To the Galloway NYC Running Club.** You make running 26.2 miles seem like a walk in the park. I'm continually motivated by the support and encouragement you share with me—and every other member of our pack. Saturday at 8 a.m.? I'm in.

• **To Myrna Blyth and the entire team at AARP Media.** Myrna, senior vice president and editorial director at AARP Media, first suggested that I write this book a few years ago. Since her early nudge, it has grown into a much bigger work than either one of us had imagined. I thank everyone at AARP for supporting the message that life can be amazing at every age, and for allowing me to help carry the banner. A very special shout-out to Jodi Lipson, director of the book division at AARP, who was a brilliant partner from start to finish; Michelle Harris, for checking facts, statistics, and quotes to make sure this book would always be held to the highest standards; Jeffrey Eagle, vice president and director of AARP Studios; and everyone on the public relations team who helped me get the powerful messages of this book out to the world.

• **To Hilary Black and the team at National Geographic.** Pinch me! I still can't believe my great luck that Hilary, my editor at National Geographic Books, saw the potential in this book, in me, and in a partnership with AARP to publish it. She has also earned a very special thank-you for giving me the space and time to come up with many titles, until together, we settled on the right one. I send my great appreciation to everyone on the National Geographic team, especially Allyson Johnson, whose edits and suggestions have been consistently thoughtful, elegant, and essential; Elisa Gibson, art director with a flair for fabulous covers and fun graphics; Nicole Miller, design production coordinator, who helped bring the pages to joyful life; and Michael O'Connor, production editor, and Elizabeth Johnson, copy editor, who made sure every *i* was dotted, as they should always be. A super-huge thank you goes to Heidi Vincent, Jessie Chirico, and Ann Day, the marketing and publicity wonder women behind the book.

• **To Andrea Galyean, editor extraordinaire with benefits.** Andrea listened, questioned, suggested, organized, proofread, and was crucial to keeping me laser-focused during the writing and editing of this book (as well as my first). Every exchange made me laugh, gave me something new to consider, and made me a better writer. I truly could not imagine attempting the next book without her ... and won't.

• **To Cynthia Cannell, my patient, brilliant agent.** Cynthia has never failed to calm, defend, support, and encourage me; and she kept me on task during the many months it took to research, write, and rewrite this book. I am grateful for Cynthia's friendship and guidance, which has made me a stronger author.

• **To my family.** Writing a book is a huge undertaking, but it would have been an even bigger challenge without the understanding, encouragement, and love of my entire family. I send a special shout-out to my sister, Carole, and mother, Pauline, for always sounding enthusiastic about the book, even after receiving yet another "What do you think of this title?" email. But my husband, Howard, and daughters, Sarah and Elizabeth, deserve nothing short of medals for their patience during the whole process. They have earned my deepest gratitude and everlasting love for their unwavering support—and for allowing me to nag the heck out of them over dinner every time I joyfully uncovered a new fact, statistic, or study about health, happiness, sleep, brain functioning, or the importance of good habits. Each fresh lecture was greeted with only a modicum of eye-rolling. They are wonderful.

• **And to my dear readers.** You know the secret to real happiness. You know that the magic happens as soon as you take that first step toward loving yourself. That's the incredible and freeing moment when everything falls into place and you truly understand that nothing can stop you. I thank each and every one of you for joining me on this incredible trip into the best years of our lives … one small step at a time.

About the Author

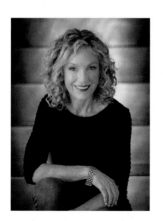

Barbara Hannah Grufferman is a nationally recognized advocate for positive living and healthy aging. Her previous book, *The Best of Everything After 50*, is a best-selling resource for women over 50. She has appeared on numerous television shows including the *Today* show, *CBS This Morning, Dr. Phil, The Doctors, The Talk,* and *Good Morning America,* as well as radio and Internet programs on NPR, Dr. Oz Sirius Radio, OWN—the Oprah Channel, and SiriusXM's Doctor Radio.

Grufferman writes regularly for HuffPost and AARP, and she hosts AARP web-based videos focusing on health, wellness, and positive aging. A recipient of the Generations of Strength Award from the National Osteoporosis Foundation, she was named the foundation's first ambassador for bone health and serves on the board of trustees. She also travels around the country to speak about the power of taking small steps toward personal transformation.

A dedicated runner and knitter, Grufferman lives in New York City with her husband and daughters—two lovely young women who have also started running, perhaps thanks to the gentle push (okay: nag) of their mother.

Illustrations Credits

Cover, PeopleImages/iStockPhoto; 2–3, kali9/Getty Images; 6, colnihko/Shutterstock; 9, Thomas Barwick/Getty Images; 14, Tetra Images/Getty Images; 21, Elnur/Getty Images; 25, stuartbur/Getty Images; 26, Andris Tkacenko/Shutterstock; 29, BJI/Blue Jean Images/Getty Images; 34, Stephen Lux/Getty Images; 37, ciud/Getty Images; 39, Dave and Les Jacobs/Getty Images; 40, flyfloor/Getty Images; 45, Tatuasha/Shutterstock; 47, Africa Studio/Shutterstock; 48, Maskot/Getty Images; 50, Alexander Raths/Shutterstock; 53, photomaru/Getty Images; 56, kaanates/Getty Images; 58, julichka/Getty Images; 59, Floortje/Getty Images; 64, wanpatsorn/Shutterstock; 67, mylisa/Shutterstock; 70, Makistock/Shutterstock; 71, matkub2499/Shutterstock; 76, Jessica Peterson/Getty Images; 80, Fotoplanner/Getty Images; 82, Lebazele/Getty Images; 85, Ilya_Starikov/Getty Images; 90, Dudaeva/Shutterstock; 94, Tom Merton/Getty Images; 96, Liliboas/Getty Images; 99, kai keisuke/Shutterstock; 100, ValentynVolkov/Getty Images; 103, Feng Yu/Shutterstock; 104, Sathit/Shutterstock; 105, atoss/Getty Images; 106, Melanie Hobson/EyeEm/Getty Images; 108, felixR/Getty Images; 111, peang/Shutterstock; 112, MarieC2/Getty Images; 114, Iurii Kachkovskyi/Shutterstock; 116, Picsfive/Shutterstock; 118, Merkushev Vasiliy/Shutterstock; 122, Lluís Real/Getty Images; 124, FabrikaCr/Getty Images; 128, Chinnasut Nhurod/Shutterstock; 129, LightField Studios/Shutterstock; 132, margouillat photo/Shutterstock; 133, eurobanks/Getty Images; 136, 58shadows/Getty Images; 139, Elya Vatel/Shutterstock; 142, dmbaker/Getty Images; 144, Ivan Masiuk/Shutterstock; 145, Enlightened Media/Shutterstock; 151, Inara Prusakova/Shutterstock; 153, dionisvero/Getty Images; 154, Katherine Fawssett/Getty Images; 156, LattaPictures/Getty Images; 158, karandaev/Getty Images; 166, addkm/Shutterstock; 168, Alain Daussin/Getty Images; 170, buradaki/Getty Images; 172, sruilk/Shutterstock; 174, GSPictures/Getty Images; 176, Gnilenkov Aleksey/Shutterstock; 179, narcisa/Getty Images; 180, eli_asenova/Getty Images; 183, scanrail/Getty Images; 185, Mehmet Hilmi Barcin/Gety Images; 191, JGI/Jamie Grill/Getty Images; 192, margostock/Getty Images; 194, Atiketta Sangasaeng/Shutterstock; 201, Africa Studio/Shutterstock; 207, zoranm/Getty Images; 208, Lev Savitskiy/Shutterstock; 209, monkeybusinessimages/Getty Images; 215, Charan Rattanasupphasiri/Shutterstock; 217, VladTeodor/Getty Images; 220, wundervisuals/Getty Images; 225, Kagenmi/Getty Images; 229, kupicoo/Getty Images; 230, hudiemm/Getty Images; 239, Nattika/Shutterstock; 244, Rawpixel/Getty Images; 249, dien/Shutterstock; 251, Eloi_Omella/Getty Images; 252, Nor Gal/Shutterstock; 255, Jeremy Bentham/Shutterstock; 258, Dave and Les Jacobs/Blend Images; 260, Ableimages/Getty Images; 264, JANIFEST/Getty Images; 267, Floortje/Getty Images; 271, _human/Getty Images; 272, Chloe Crespi Photography/Getty Images; 274, Imo/Getty Images; 275, petrenkod/Getty Images; 277, John Warburton-Lee/Getty Images; 279, n_defender/Shutterstock 286, Howard Steven Grufferman; back cover (LE), Morsa Images/Getty Images; (LE CT), SrdjanPav/Getty Images; (RT CT), a_namenko/Getty Images; (RT), tonivaver/Getty Images.

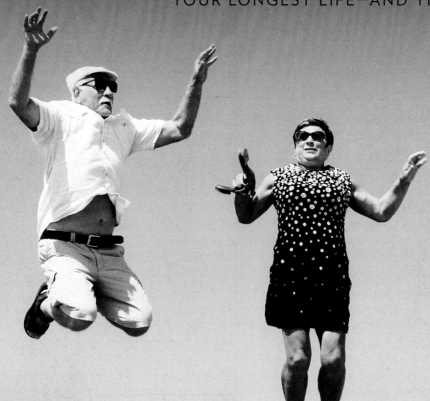
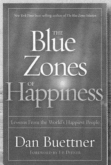
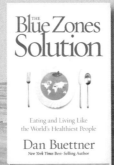
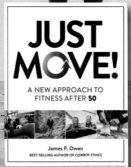
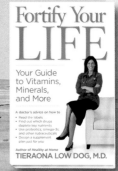
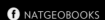 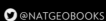
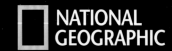